QuickTime ECG

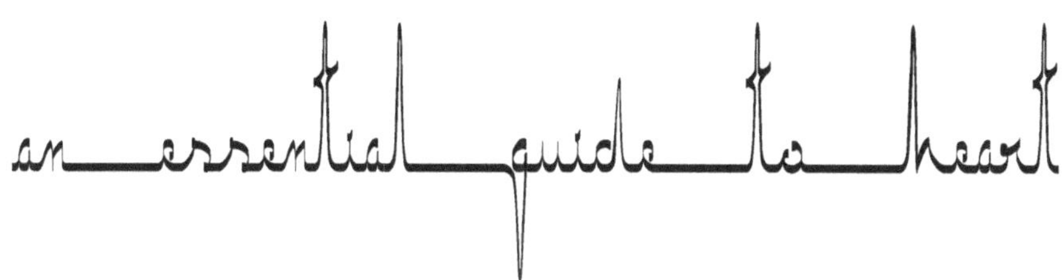

Dr. B. Sen, MD

Associate Professor
Department of Practice of Medicine
West Bengal University of Health Sciences

Dedicated

In the memory of my teacher who taught to look at heart

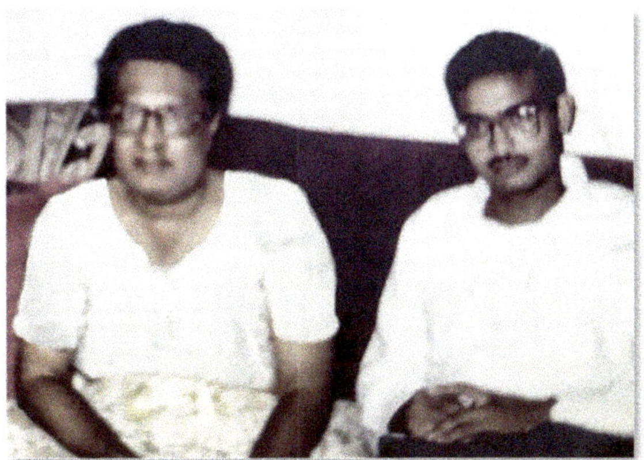

Dr. Rajat Mahapatra, DM (Cardiology), ABIM, FACA, FICA
Ex-Associate Professor: Internal Medicine, Texas State University, USA

&

my father for my all-good sides

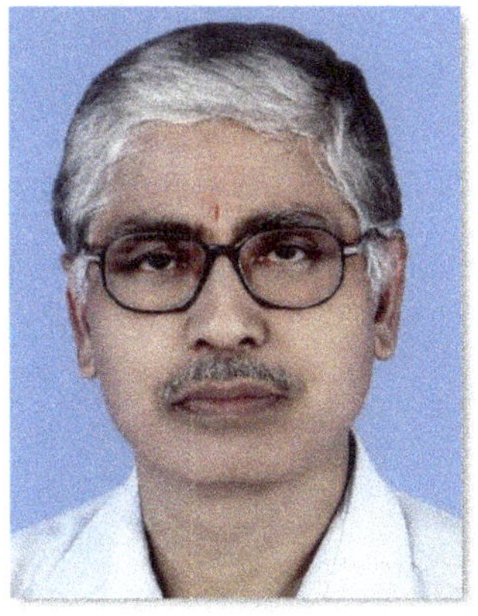

Mr. Rabindra Nath Sen, BSc, LLB

Contents

Preface

With the infiltration of advanced instruments in medical field, clinical acumen with thousands of years of experience is gradually fading. But no instrument can replace clinical acumen ever! Investigation report still mentions "... please correlate clinically ...," which proves all.

ECG, an aged health instrument based on electro-physics imparting its stake since 1887 but still no younger competitor! Rather with the advancement of the instrument, now part of clinical examination like stethoscope or pulse-oximeter.

There is plethora of books on ECG, and every book is worthy for its approach with similar or different notes. In this book, author tried to loosen the knots of fear generally found in the mind of a sophomore, to draw interest by adding several illustrations, taste of humor to make it interesting and nurture intuition so engaging.

To an expert it may be 'Just another book', but I request them to go through the book and taste the different flavor that they may miss in other books. It is prepared to make them nostalgic! I request, proficient medical fraternity to help me find the darker side of the book by giving essential constructive inputs, for which I will always be indebted.

I express my sincerest gratitude to my first teachers, my parents; my cardiology teacher Dr. R. K. Mahapatra; and the patients who suffer my nagging with a smile to take at times serial ECGs for academic purposes. This is the best place to beg pardon to my wife Dr. Usha Sen who sacrificed a lot swapping many family responsibilities from me. I also say sorry to my son Bisweswar, not giving him much of myself, I love you.

My work will be fruitful, if the reader gains an acumen on ECG with ease and save suffering humanity in the high time of need.

Place   : Kolkata, INDIA
Date   : 24.10.2023

Dr. Biswarup Sen, MD
Practice of Medicine (Hom.)
doctor_sen@rediffmail.com

🫀Get Set Go ....

Ensure enough glucose supply to your brain …. take a deep breath ….
FREE your mind …. let us start the wonderful journey to the heart.

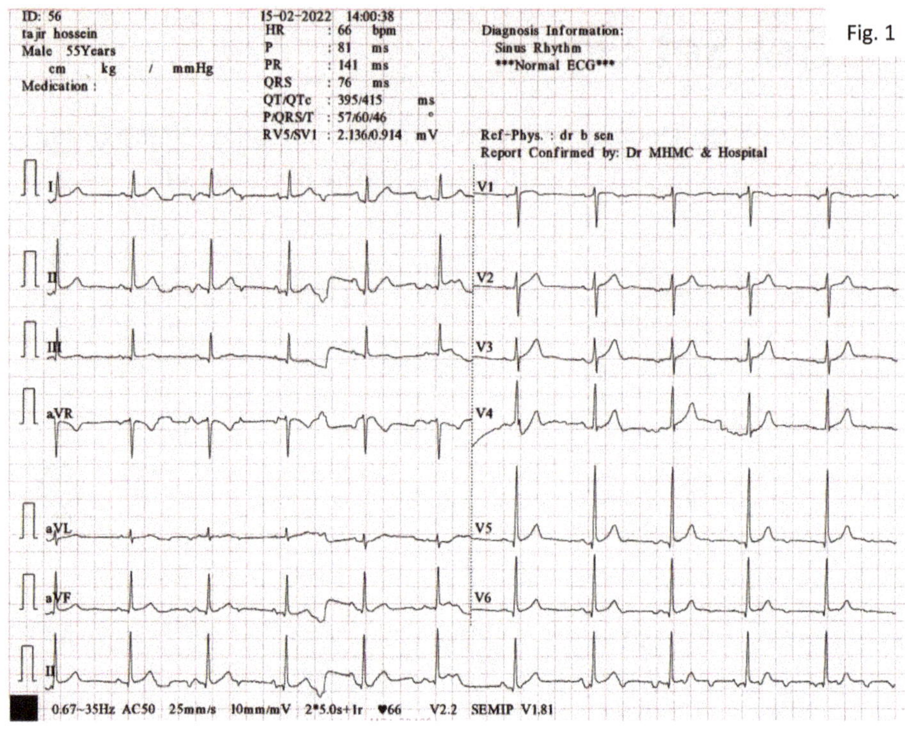

STATUTORY WARNING

ECG (EKG) is nothing but the 'summation vector' of electrical events interpreted on graph paper in a specialized and standardized way. So, in some conditions though rare, a very abnormal heart (electronically at least) may produce normal ECG pattern and vice versa.

So, ECG is a tool, which must be confirmed by clinical and further investigatory procedures – and nothing is absolute 😢.

Do not be 💔! Most of the cases **we shall** 💥 !

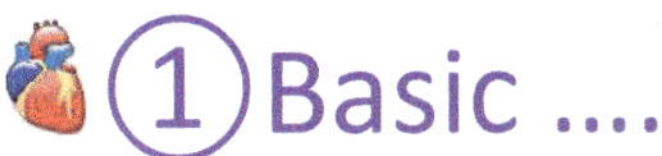 ① Basic ....

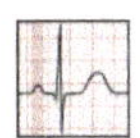

Heart – the power generator

At resting state, cardiac cells are electronically 'polarized;' i.e., the cell interior is negatively charged in respect to the outside.

'Depolarization' occurs when the cells lose internal electro-negativity.

Depolarization propagates from one cell to another; thus, an electrical depolarizing current is formed, which transmitted to entire heart.

After completion of depolarization, cardiac cells restore to their resting (negative) polarity by 'repolarization.'

Both 'depolarization' and 'repolarization' are detected by electrodes of ECG-machine placed on surface of the body as if CCTV watching the electrical events of the heart from various angles and perspectives.

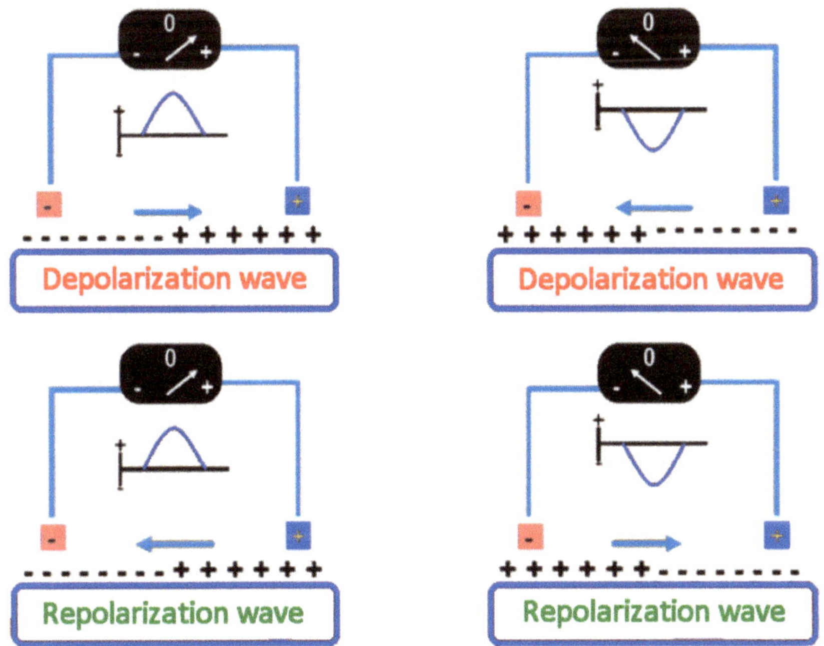

Fig. 2

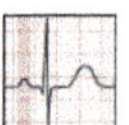

Electrical architecture of Heart

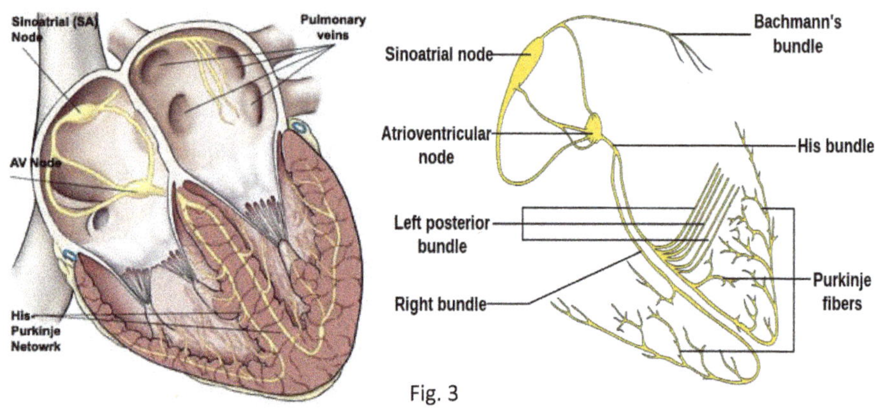

Fig. 3

> **Pacemaker cells**: the King - generator of electricity
> Small cells having capacity to depolarize spontaneously ["Anahata chakra" (*Sans.*) = generate impulse without any input!] till death. Rate is determined by internal circuitry and external neurohormonal stimulus. Dominant pacemaker cells located at the superior part of the right atrium named sinoatrial/sinus/SA node, governs whole heart to beat normally @ 60-100 bpm.

> **Conducting path**: the wire/highway via which electricity passes
> Long thin cells having plenty of gap junctions, thus swiftly conduct the flow to the distant regions of the heart.

> **Myocardial cells**: the slave – contracts on electrical whip
> The effector organ and largest part contains plenty of contractile tissue, which effectively contracts, on stimulation; flow slowly propagates throughout the heart.

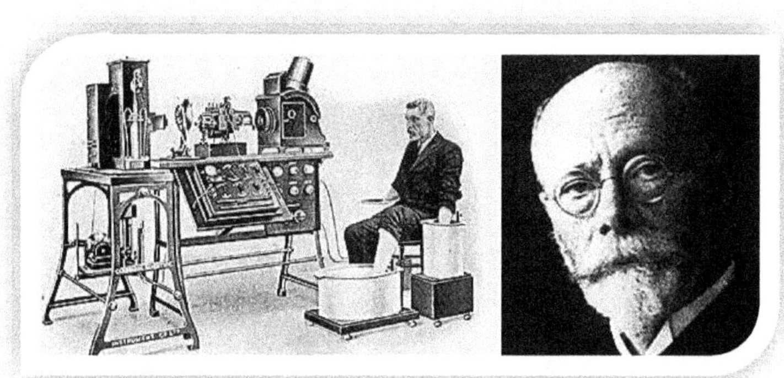

Sir William Einthoven – inventing the first electrocardiogram

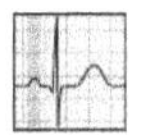 # Time and Tide

The current plotted on a universally standardized ECG, principally reflects the electrical activity of dominant myocardium as the other events are usually electrically subtle enough not to be caught by.

Like any other tide it too has three major components –
1. DURATION (second)
2. AMPLITUDE (millivolts)
3. CONFIGURATION

There is a motor that rotates at a specific speed, rolling the standardized graph paper and a pointer marker fixed with voltmeter that deflects with flow of current; put mark on moving graph paper; scribing the ECG.

The graph paper contains large dark squares (5x5 mm^2), which are subdivided into five small faint squares (1x1 mm^2).

The horizontal axis measures time: the motor rotates at such a speed that each small square corresponds to 0.04 second, and the large one (0.04 sec x 5 small squares) to 0.2 second.

The vertical axis measures voltage: standardized as, two large squares correspond to 1 millivolt (mV), so each small square 0.1 mV.

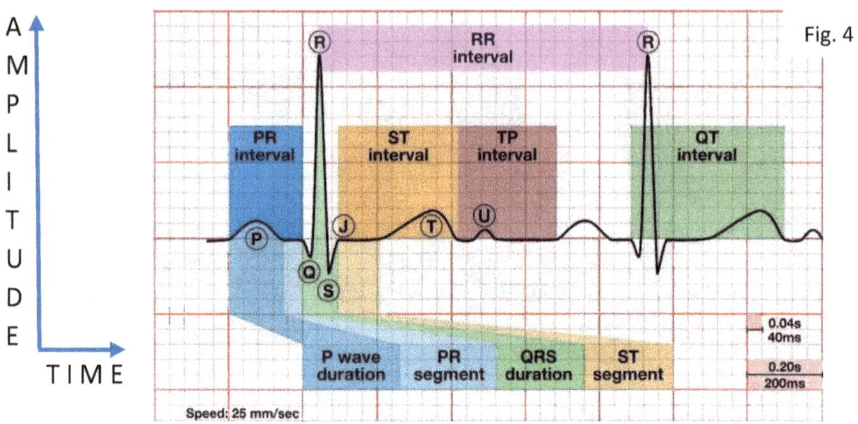

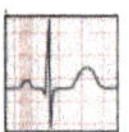

Architecture of the current

ELECTRICAL EVENT leads to MECHANICAL EVENT
ELECTRICAL EVENT is faster than MECHANICAL EVENT

Every cell in the heart has the potential to initiate pace-making but the highest rate generator rules the rest. So, normally the electrical cycle of the heart starts with the firing of the 'King' pacemaker, i.e., SA node. The current depolarization spreads eccentrically to atrial myocardium, which is called ATRIAL DEPOLARIZATION, scribed as 'P wave.'

As SA node is situated at the superior part of the right atrium, the right atrium depolarizes earlier than the left atrium and finishes earlier as well. So, the first part of the 'P wave' predominantly represents the depolarization of the right atrium and the last part of the left atrium.

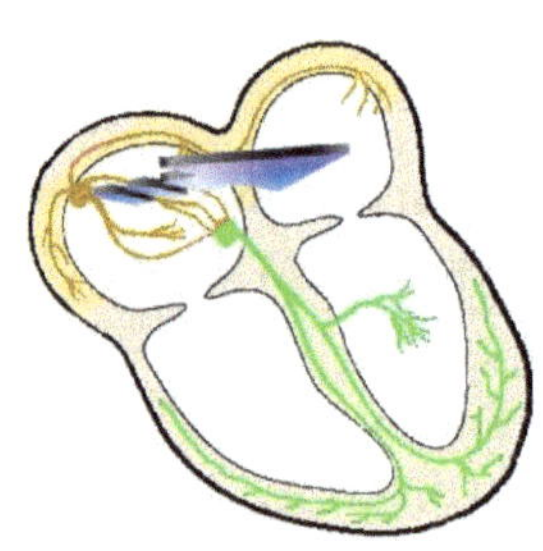

Fig. 5

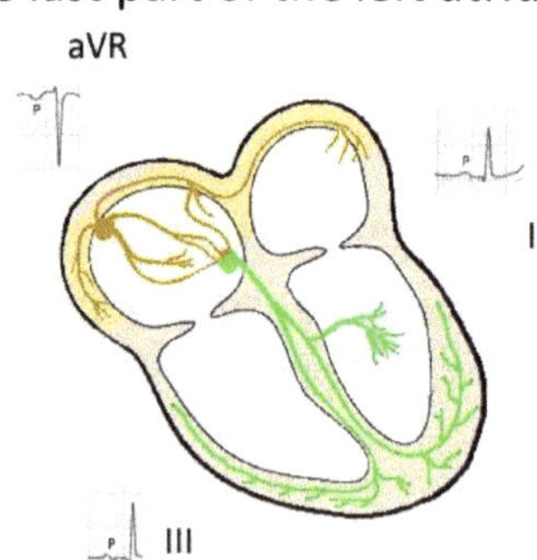

Following the atrial depolarization, ECG becomes electrically silent. Healthy heart has a 'toll-plaza' i.e., electrical window named 'Atrioventricular/AV node' at the junction of the atria and ventricles. Only through that, the current can pass but with a delay in conduction from atria to ventricles. This **crucial pause** (PR segment) helps atria to pour all collected blood to ventricles.

Like the SA node, AV node too is determined by internal circuitry and external neurohormonal stimulus – autonomic nervous system, especially vagus. Vagal stimulation further slows down the conduction and on the contrary sympathetic stimulation accelerates it.

Following the toll plaza there should be an expressway. Yes! here also no exception. As soon as the depolarization current leaves the AV node, it comes out swiftly to ventricles via specialized conduction pathway. The pathway consists of three major parts (Page 4, Fig. 3):

1. Bundle of His (Wilhelm His Jr.)
2. Bundle branches (right and left)
3. Purkinje fibers (Jan Evangelista P.)

Bundle of His is truly short, just after the exit from AV node, it divides into right bundle branch (RBB) and left bundle branch (LBB). The RBB supplies the current to the right side of interventricular septum (IVS) all the way to the apex of right ventricle. The LBB divides into three major fascicles:

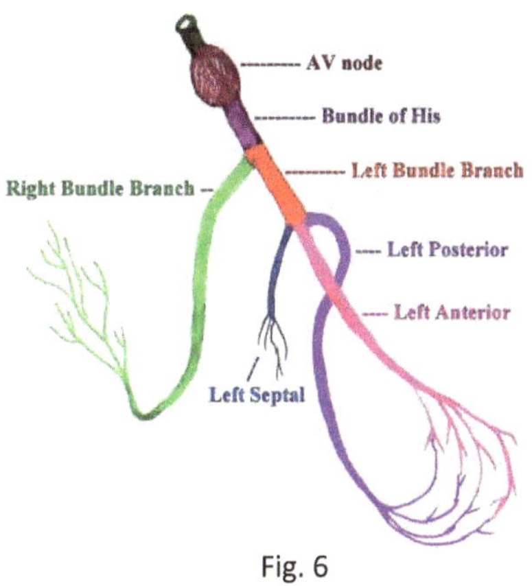

Fig. 6

1. Anterior : Anterior wall of the left ventricle
2. Posterior: Posterior wall of the left ventricle
3. Septal   : Interventricular septum (IVS), direction left to right

Bundle branches break in innumerable small Purkinje fibers, which delivers the current to the myocardial cells.

Ventricular depolarization causes ventricular systole, which is scribed on ECG as large deflection as '**QRS complex**' (Page 6, Fig. 4). As the ventricles have much larger muscle mass than the atria, the amplitude of the QRS complex is much larger and sharper than that of 'P wave.'

'**QRS complex**' has several distinct components which have particular significance too. As the architecture of the QRS complex varies largely, a standardized nomenclature introduced as follows (Page 6, Fig. 4):

1. If the first deflection is downward, it is called a 'Q wave.'
2. First upward deflection is called an 'R wave,' whether it is preceded. by Q wave or not.
3. Any deflection below the baseline following an R wave is called an 'S wave,' whether there is a preceding Q wave or not.
4. If there is a second upward deflection, called R'(R-prime).
5. If the whole complex has only one downward deflection, call 'QS wave.'

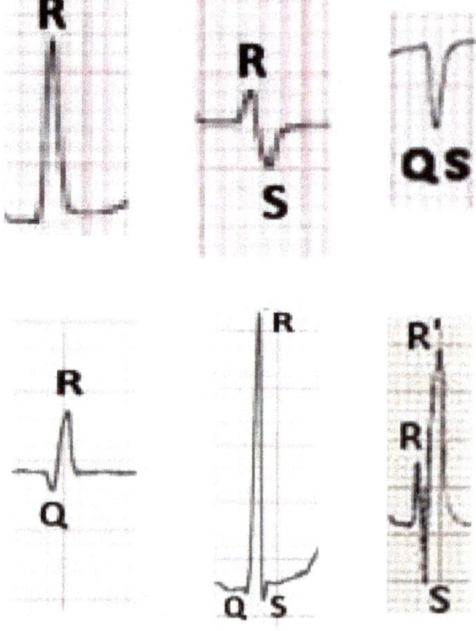

Fig. 7

The first part of the QRS complex denotes depolarization of IVS by the septal fascicle of the LBB scribes 'Q wave.' Both ventricles then depolarize almost simultaneously and scribes 'R wave,' though the leading impact on ECG is clearly produced by the left ventricular activation having 2.5 times more muscle mass. 'S wave' scribed due to the depolarization of the uppermost part of the ventricles.

Following the depolarization of myocardial cells; there is a short refractory period scribed on ECG as 'ST-segment,' during this time cells cannot be re-stimulated.

To regain the resting phase, cells start to 'repolarize' comparatively slowly by restoring electronegativity inside; thus, prepared to sense further stimulation. Atrial repolarization wave is too weak to scribe any impression on ECG as it also buried under mighty QRS complex; ventricular repolarization wave is scribed like a hump on ECG as 'T wave,' as it takes longer time.

Measuring the QT-interval, *never rely on the auto-interpretation by ECG-machine*; prime drawback of auto-interpretation which may include discrete U waves in calculations, leads to misleadingly high values. So, Measure from the Q wave to the juncture of the T wave major slope with the isoelectric line.

Fig. 8

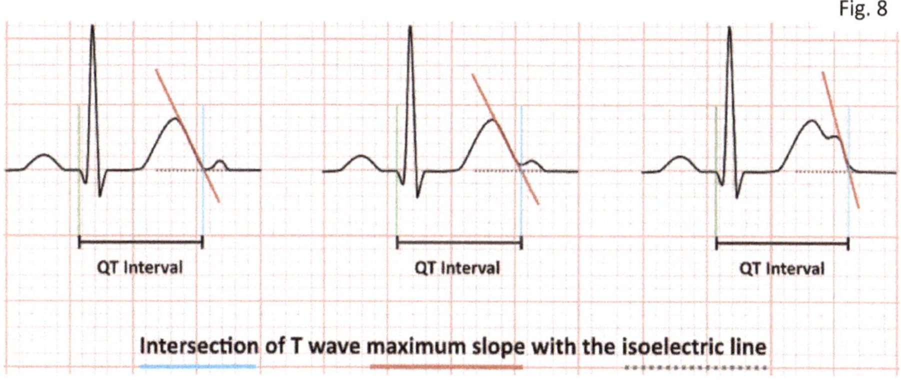

A segment is a straight line connecting two waves, whereas an interval at least one wave combined with the connecting straight line mostly.

As the resultant *summation vector* of electrical wave progresses from one point to another, sensed by the electrodes placed at various parts on the surface of the body. The wave of depolarization (inner state of cells become positive) moving towards a positive electrode scribe positive deflection and away from a positive electrode scribe negative deflection. Equally, the wave of depolarization moving towards a positive electrode scribe positive deflection and away from a positive electrode scribe negative deflection (Page 3, Fig. 2). It is worth noticing that, when a depolarizing wave moves perpendicularly to a positive electrode, it scribes biphasic wave. On these basics, now we just put cameras (leads) on various positions on the body surface surrounding heart.

Fig. 9

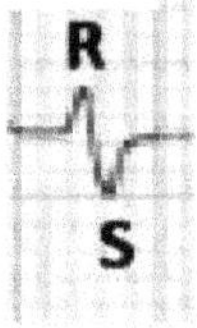

As a standard safety procedure, we use at least twelve cameras to investigate what is going in the heart electrically to ascertain the suspect, i.e., 12-lead ECG. To get the picture in twelve cameras, we need 4 limb (2 placed on arms and 2 on legs) and 6* precordial electrodes; these 10 electrodes one of which use as ground, virtually serve as 12 cameras included as 3 standard limb leads and 3 augmented limb leads.

The **limb leads** are planted to watch the heart on frontal plane by putting electrodes on all four limbs. The frontal plane can now be projected as a big circle superimposed on the body. These leads scribe the waves moving superior to inferior and side by side.

As stated, leads are nothing but cameras which catch the transit of electrical wave of heart, so placed in specific *'angle of orientation (AO).'*

Standard limb leads:

1. Lead-I : Left arm positive, right arm negative   → AO = +0°.
2. Lead-II : Both legs positive, right arm negative → AO = +60°.
3. Lead-III: Both legs positive, left arm negative   → AO = +120°.

Augmented limb leads:

4. aVR: Right arm positive, other limbs negative → AO = -150°.
5. aVL: Left arm positive, other limbs negative   → AO = -30°.
6. aVF: Both legs positive, both arms negative   → AO = +90°.

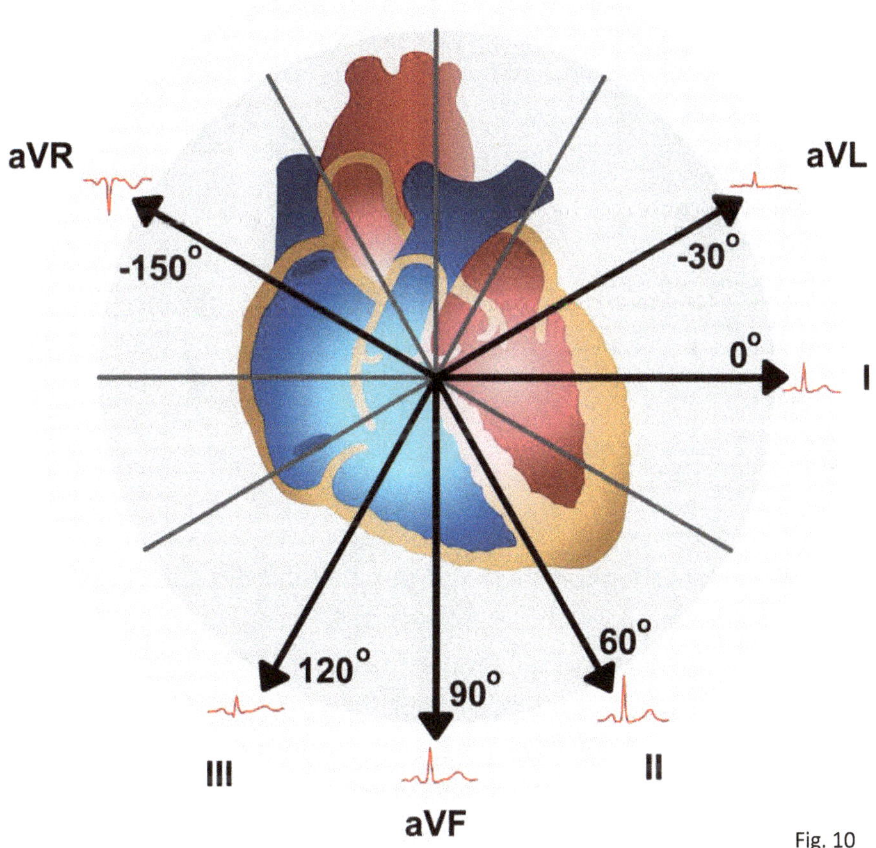

Fig. 10

Precordial **leads** are planted to watch the heart on horizontal plane. These leads scribe the waves moving anterior to posterior. Here all six precordial leads are taken as positive electrode individually and whole body taken as ground. Placement of precordial leads are as follows:

1. V_1 : Right sternal border, 4th intercostal space
2. V_2 : Left sternal border, 4th intercostal space
3. V_3 : Placed between V_2 & V_4
4. V_4 : Left midclavicular line, 5th intercostal space
5. V_5 : Left anterior axillary line, 5th intercostal space (between V_4-V_6)
6. V_6 : Left midaxillary line, 5th intercostal space

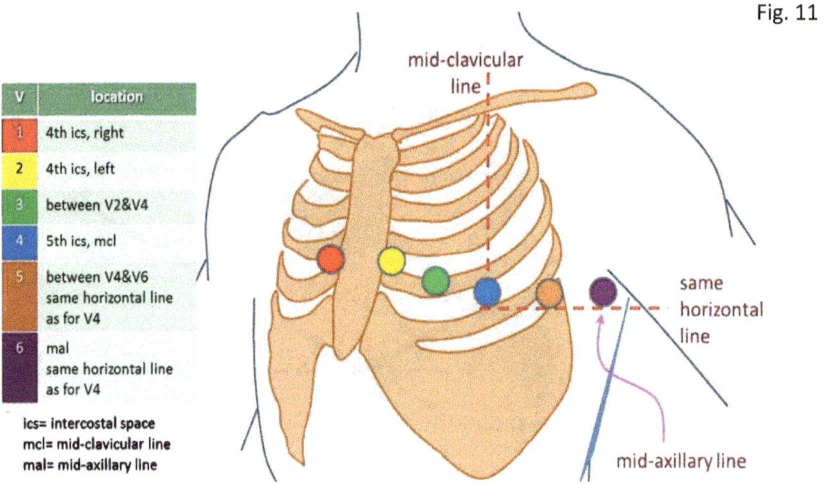

Fig. 11

Now, these leads look at the heart in particular directions assigned to them positionally. As the right ventricle lies antero-medially, left ventricle lies postero-laterally; V_1 lies just over the right ventricle, V_2, V_3 over interventricular septum, V_4 over the apex and V_5, V_6 over lateral part of left ventricle. Briefly,

Anterior	: V_2, V_3, V_4
Left lateral	: I, aVL, V_5, V_6
Inferior	: II, III, aVF
Right ventricular	: aVR, V_1

♥ Conventional 12-lead ECG

For smooth entertainment of a car race needs some prerequisites. As,

♥ Road condition, and where to pause / accelerate – pathway & car.

♥ Proper installation of cameras, to catch every lap – the leads in the exact position (here leads only record the average flow of wave).

First and small bump, state highway – P wave:

Atrial depolarization begins at SA node which is situated in the high and upper right corner of the right atrium, wave spreading from right atrium to left atrium. The resultant summation vector (henceforth will be called as 'vector') flows a little downward and to the left.

aVL, I, II and aVF are the leads, which view the wave of atrial depolarization moving towards them, scribe positive deflection on the ECG paper; Lead III positioned perpendicular to the wave – scribes a biphasic pattern. aVR being the remaining lead on frontal plane, views the wave to go away from it, scribe negative deflection. In horizontal plane, left lateral leads i.e., V_5, V_6 views same as I, aVL scribe positive deflection. V_1 views as lead III, so biphasic. Atria being small thin walled, can generate low voltage; so, the amplitude normally does not exceed 0.25 mV (2½ small squares from baseline in any leads). Vector of atrial depolarization ranges as wide as +0° to +70° and of moderate speed; so, biphasic wave cannot be always true to lead II or V_1.

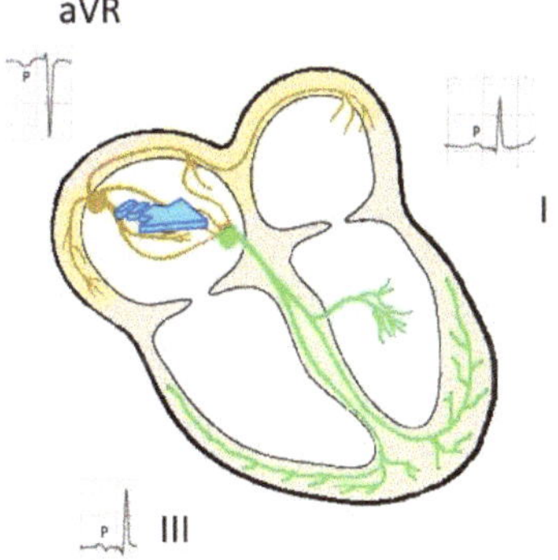

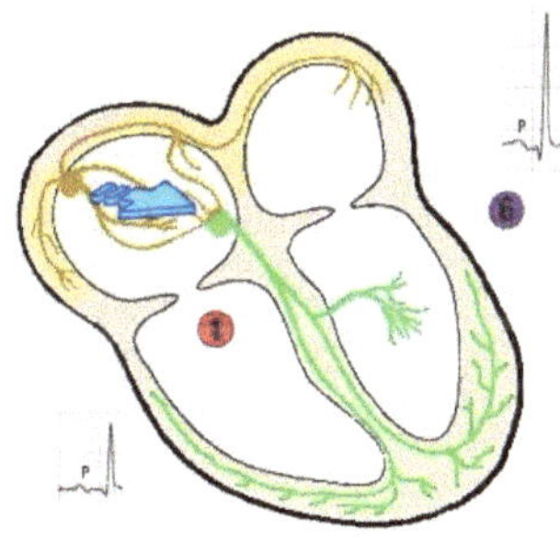

Fig. 12

Let us take a break, toll plaza – PR segment:
It represents the time from the end of atrial depolarization to the beginning of ventricular depolarization, it denotes the time of **crucial pause** at AV junction; so that the atria can pour most blood to ventricles. ECG shows no undulation due to virtually halted electrical activity.

PR-interval represents the time from the beginning of the atrial depolarization to the beginning of the ventricular depolarization. It normally times 0.12 to 0.2 seconds, i.e., between 3 to 5 small squares.

Expressway, swift away – QRS complex:
After the AV node, the wave of depolarization reached a fast-conducting pathway and produces the QRS complex.

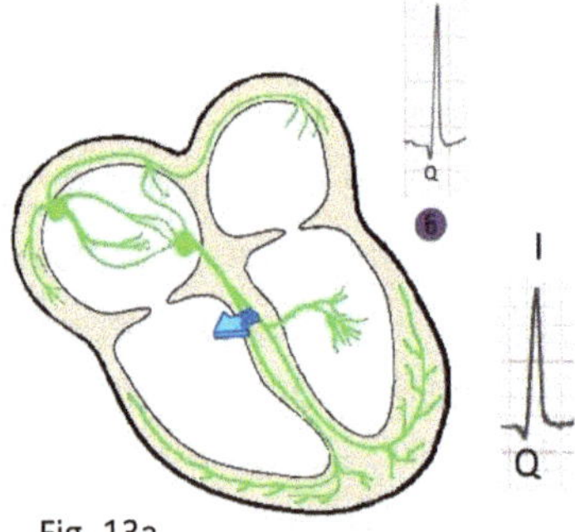

Fig. 13a

The interventricular septum is first depolarized by the septal fascicle of the LBB scribes 'Q wave.' As small area depolarizes, impression of the event may not be found always, if present it scribes a small negative (downward) deflection, normally of <0.1mV on left sided leads and occasionally on inferior leads.

Both ventricles then depolarize almost simultaneously due to fastest conducting pathway scribes positive (upward) deflection as 'R wave'. Though the leading impact on ECG is clearly produced by the left

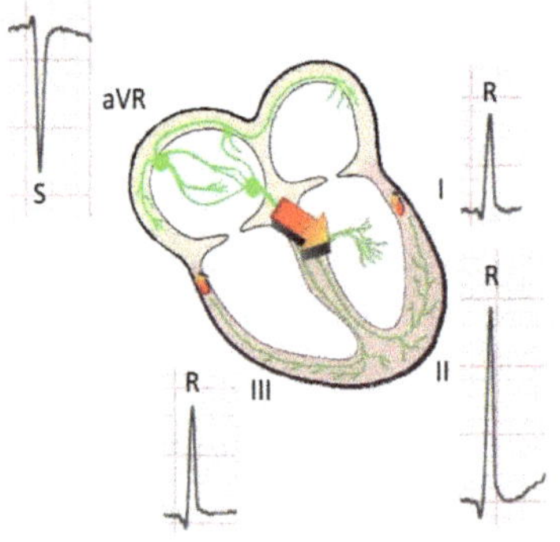

Fig. 13b

ventricular repolarization having almost three times myocardial mass. Vector of ventricular depolarization ranges as wide as +0° to +90°. 'S wave' scribed due to the depolarization of the uppermost part of the ventricles. So, in the frontal plane long upward R waves scribe in left lateral and inferior leads but as the wave going away rapidly form aVR, deep S waves.

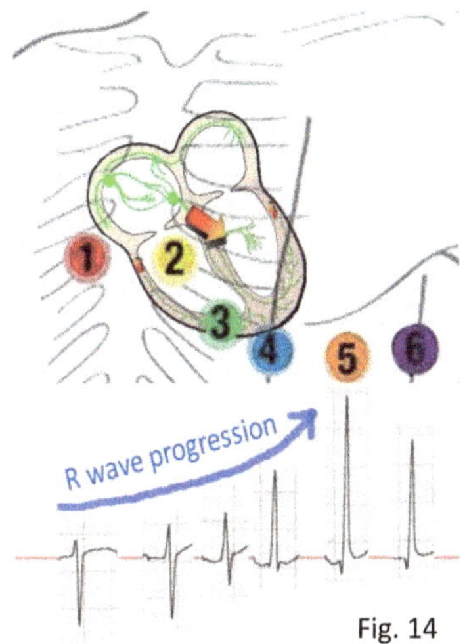

Fig. 14

Similarly, in horizontal plane, precordial lead V_1 and V_2 superimpose right ventricle, so usually scribes a deep 'S wave' as the wave is moving away from it; on contrary, V_5 and V_6 superimpose left ventricle, scribe tall positive R waves. V_3 and V_4 overlies in between them, scribe *'biphasic'* wave, i.e., 'R wave' and 'S wave' of nearly equal amplitude. It is notable that, from right to left, the gradual deepening of 'S wave' replaced by the upshoot of the 'R wave;' this is called '***R wave progression***.'

Practically this progression seen V_1 to V_5 and V_6 is usually have smaller 'R' than V_5. The amplitude is much higher than atrial depolarization, as ventricles have much more myocardial mass. QRS interval is the duration of the 'QRS complex,' normally it ranges 0.06 to 0.1 seconds.

Following the depolarization of myocardial cells; there is a short refractory period scribed as horizontal or slight upsloping on ECG as 'ST-segment' in almost all leads. It denotes the time from the end of ventricular depolarization to the start of ventricular repolarization.

End of journey, refueling – T wave:
It denotes the ventricular repolarization, which is an active process, requires affluent energy to run the 'voltage gated' pumps. So, this part is most vulnerable to all sorts of intra / extra-cardiac stimuli and thus widely differing in kind.

In a normal heart, repolarization usually begins in the area depolarized last, and travel backward almost following the way of depolarization. As both waves follow almost the same route but opposite direction and being electrically opposite, both scribe similar deflections on ECG.

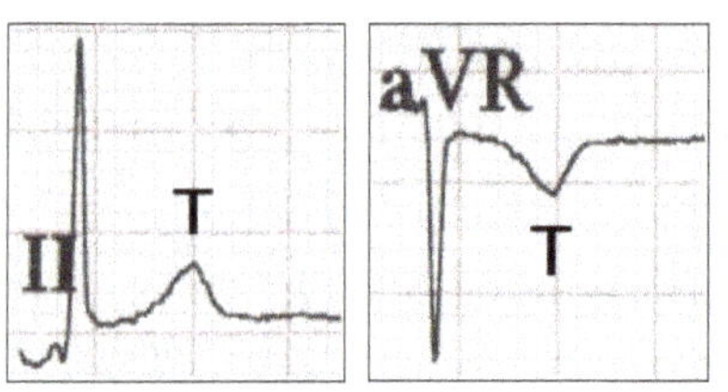

Fig. 15

So, naturally we find positive 'T waves' in leads with tall 'R waves' and negative 'T waves' with deep 'S waves.' The height of the normal 'T wave' is 1/3rd to 2/3rd of the preceding 'R wave'.

QT-interval represents the time from the beginning of ventricular depolarization to the end of ventricular repolarization, thus denotes all the electrical events of the ventricle. Duration of the QT-interval is inversely proportionate to the heart rate. So, if heart rate goes up, QT-interval shortened and vice-versa. QT-interval covers 40% of the time of entire normal cardiac cycle measured as R-R interval (Page 6, Fig. 4).

♥ Axis of the heart

'Similia Similibus Curentur' – 'Picking a thorn is easier by a similar thorn.' To easily comprehend the axis, QRS complex is the best part to look at. Instantaneous vectors, those scribe in ECG is nothing but the summation of the innumerable small vectors of ventricular depolarization and repolarization.

Beginning with the septal depolarization towards right (Page 13, Fig. 13a) the sequential vectors gradually pulled towards left (Page 13, Fig. 13b), somewhat *anti-clockwise* by the mightier left ventricular mass. Now, the summation of the instantaneous vectors is known as '**mean vector**.' The direction of the mean vector is called the '**mean electrical axis**,' henceforth will be called as '**axis**.'

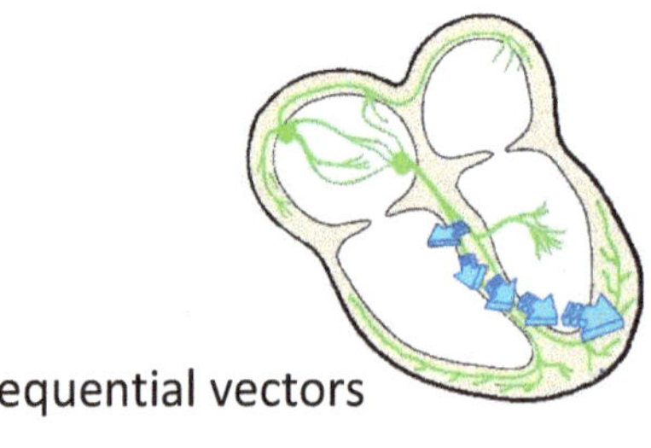

Sequential vectors

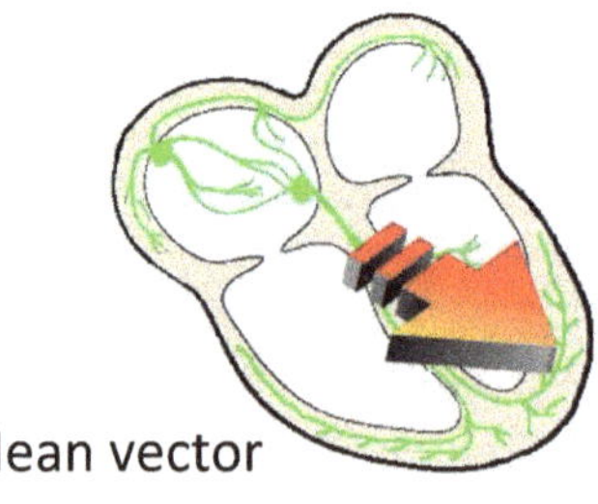

Mean vector

Fig. 16

As mean ventricular depolarization vector points antero-inferiorly and to the left, reflecting the mean direction of the current flow during entire ventricle depolarization.

Normal QRS axis is between +0∘ to +90∘ (however some cardiologist extended the range as -30∘ to +90∘ even up to +100∘). Now, as at +0∘, lead I and at +90∘, lead aVF look at, and both being situated perpendicular to each other; so, if in lead I & aVF 'QRS complex' predominantly found positive, then the axis of the heart is normal (Page 11, Fig. 9). On contrary if in both I & aVF predominantly not found positive or rather negative, then the axis is not normal.

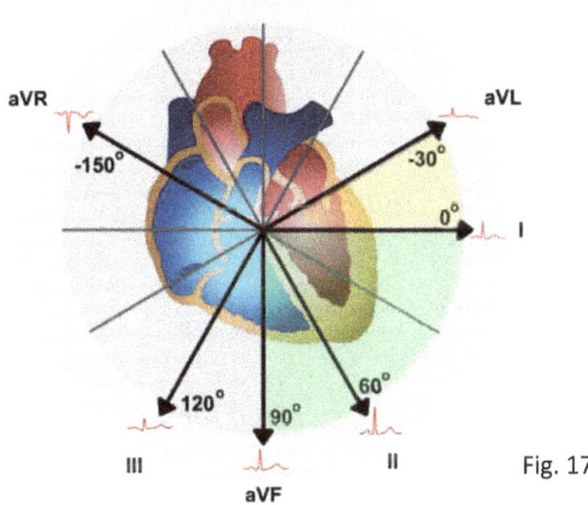

Fig. 17

A near precise angle of mean axis can be possible, we need to look at the limb leads, where the QRS complex is nearly 'biphasic' or 'flat (isoelectric);' the axis is then surely pass near or exactly perpendicular to the limb. But it only assures though which line the mean vector passes, it may be of either side, e.g., if 'biphasic' QRS found in lead aVF, then current passes exactly through lead I, but cannot confirm whether it is towards lead I or away from it. Now to confirm that, in this case we need to look at lead I – if towards it, positive else negative, and so on.

In nutshell, axis can be elicited simply looking at the different limb leads keeping the simple thing in mind, toward is upward, away is downward.

Normal 'P wave' axis is between **+0° to +70°** (**+0° to +90° in children**). 'T wave' axis is variable but approximates with a diversion ranging 50° to 60° of the QRS axis, beyond that is abnormal.

Let us try the axes of P wave, QRS complex and T wave for the ECG:

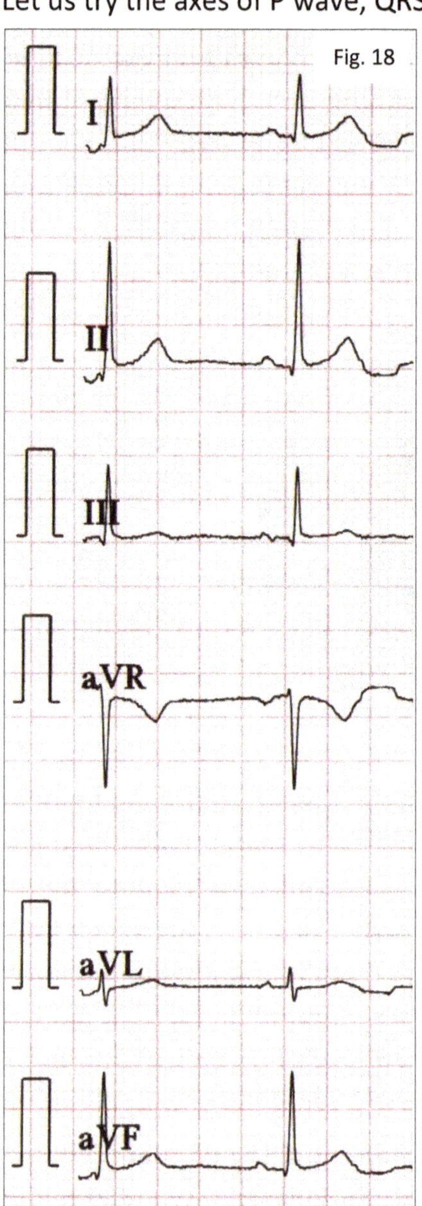

Fig. 18

P wave: In lead III 'P wave' is biphasic, so its axis is moving perpendicular to lead III is either +30° or -150°; now as the 'P wave' in lead II is positive, so the axis is positive and +30°.

QRS complex: In lead aVL 'P wave' is biphasic, so its axis is moving perpendicular to lead aVL is either +60° or -120°; now as the 'QRS complex' in lead II is positive, so the axis is positive and +60°, which is directing lead II.

T wave: 'T wave' found *flat* in lead III, so its axis is moving perpendicular to lead III is either +30° or -150°; now as the 'T wave' in lead II is tall positive, so the axis is positive and +30°, which is within the diversion range of 'QRS complex' too.

☺ Aging of Axis!

Frontal axis of QRS complex is rightward in newborns (Right ventricle relatively larger) and gradually become vertical during childhood and wind further leftward as the LV gradually increases its bulk. QRS is almost parallel to anatomical base to apex axis of heart. Axis more vertical in thin than heavy persons.

🫀②Might is right

Mightier pull all towards its interest, including more power. Heart is no exception!

It became bigger by two means; one is by exercising more it increases its muscle mass like a bodybuilder and another is by flabby dilatation like Sumo wrestler, though it is an oversimplification.

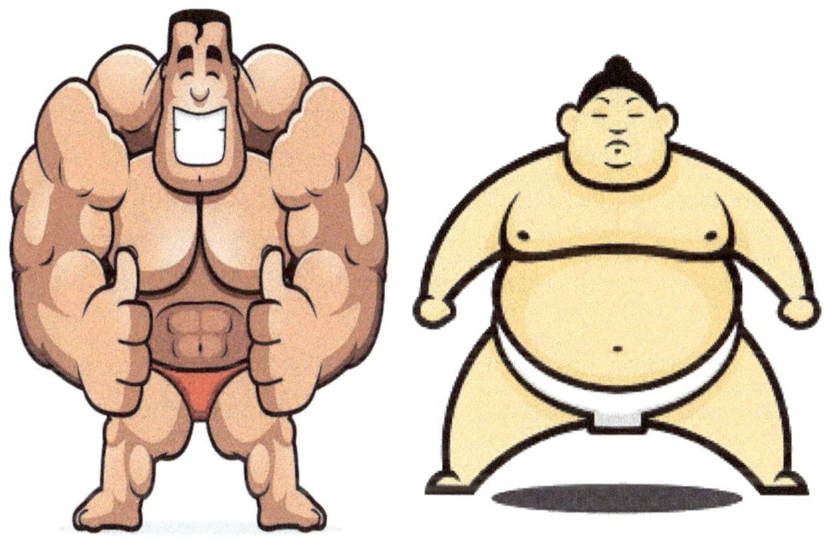

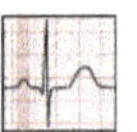 # Hypertrophy [Hyper (Gk.) = increase + tropho (Gk.) = nutrition]

Hypertrophy of heart is nothing but the increased myocardial mass due to exercise/weightlifting for long time, i.e., effect of '***pressure overload***' to the respective chamber(s), where for long-time (chronic) heart must exercise against increased resistance, as found in the patients with outflow obstructions like AS, HOCM, etc., and/or increased peripheral resistance (hypertension).

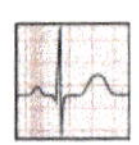 # Enlargement

Enlargement is the dilation of the respective chamber(s) of the heart usually due to sudden flooding of the blood, where it gets almost no time to cope with such 'volume overload' and eventually dilate to accommodate the increased amount of blood in the patients with especially regurgitant type of valvular lesions like AR, MR.

Both hypertrophy and enlargement often coexist to cope with the demand and Alas! ECG is not so clever to distinguish between them.

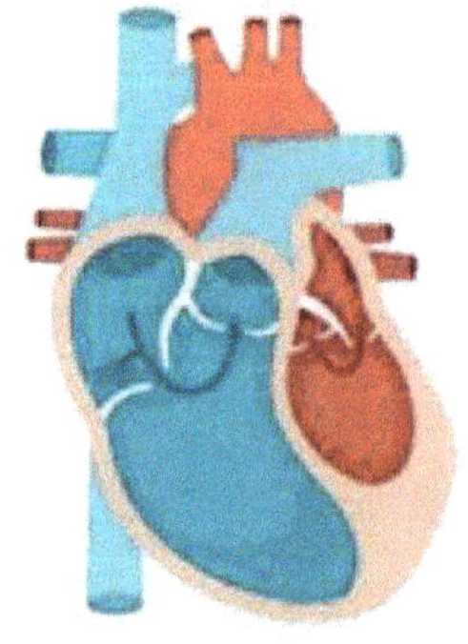
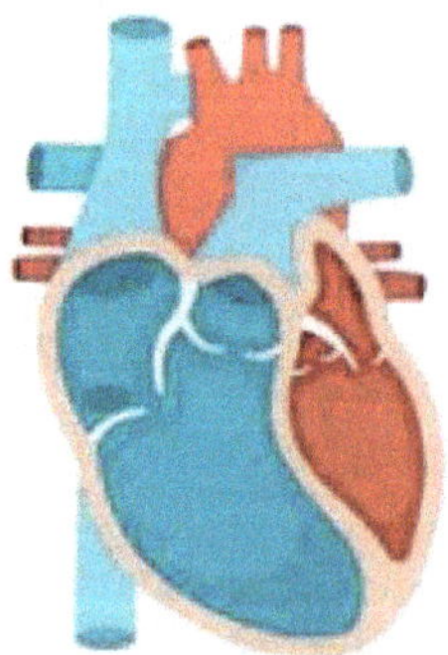
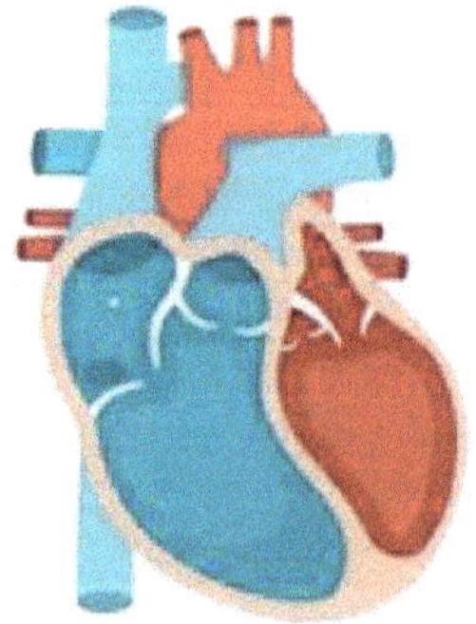

Fig. 19

Thinks to keep in mind,

1. The larger the area – longer time takes to electrify.

    – increase duration.

2. More myocardium – higher voltage generation

    – increase. of amplitude.

3. Mightier attracts power – mean vector flex toward larger side.

    – shifting of axis to mightier side.

♥ ATRIAL ENLARGEMENT (hypertrophy)

'P wave' represents atrial depolarization, due to enlargement of atria changes occur in duration, amplitude, and architecture. It is normally < 0.12 seconds in duration and largest deflection either positive or negative ≤ 2.5 mm. The first part of 'P wave' represents right atrium and last part represents left atrium as right side depolarizes first.

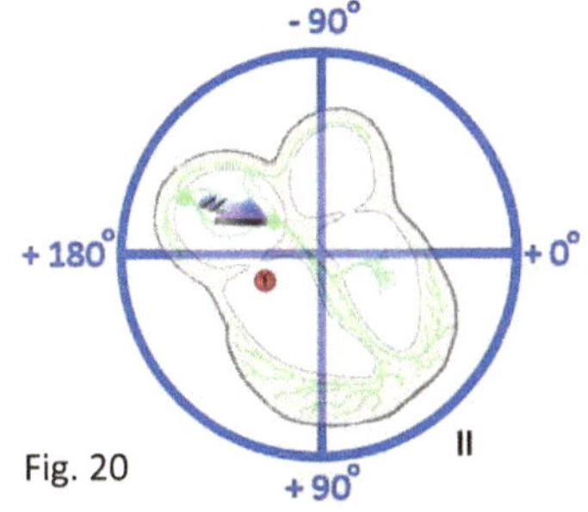

Fig. 20

We can get all the required information to judge the atrial enlargement from lead II being near parallel and V_1 being perpendicular to it, so biphasic allowing easy separation of the right and left atrial components.

RIGHT ATRIAL ENLARGEMENT

Amplitude of the first part of the 'P wave' became taller (> 2.5 mm) at least one of the inferior leads, width change buried under the last part of the 'P wave' which denotes left atrial origin. 'P wave' axis too moves towards the dominating right side sometimes even beyond +90°. So, tallest 'P wave' can be found then in aVF or even III, instead of II. The *peaking* of first part of 'P wave' is called '**P Pulmonale**' as the right atrial enlargement is usually happened due to chronic obstructive pulmonary disease; other causes are, normal variant (vertical heart, small bodily habitus, etc.), congenital heart disease (e.g., Fallot's tetralogy, pulmonic stenosis, Eisenmenger's syndrome, tricuspid atresia), pulmonary embolism (PE) and secondary to left atrial enlargement (30%).

LEFT ATRIAL ENLARGEMENT

When enlarges, duration of the 'P wave' increase as being the end-part and there is isoelectric line after, terminal portion must be > 0.04 second. The amplitude of the last part of the 'P wave' must drop > 1 mm below the isoelectric line and 40 ms wide in lead V_1. ECG scribe *notched P* and is called '**P Mitrale**' as it usually happens due to left atrial dilation and hypertrophy following mitral regurgitation.

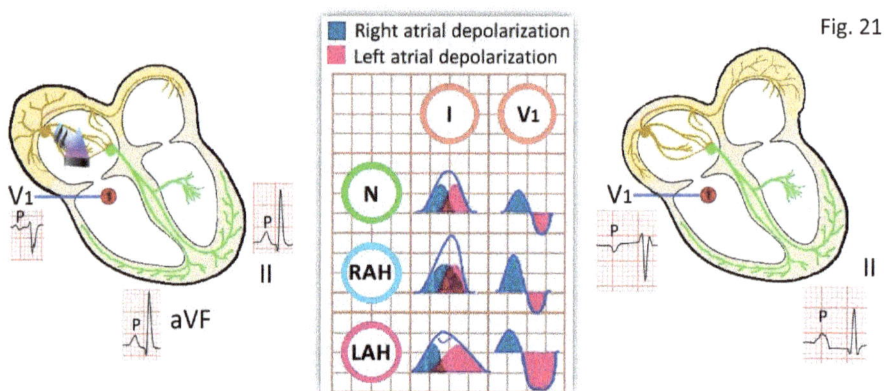

♥ VENTRICULAR HYPERTROPHY (enlargement)

'QRS complex' represents ventricular depolarization; due to hypertrophy of ventricles, changes occur in amplitude mainly but changes in duration are negligible. In normal adults, the left ventricle is 2.5 times thicker than the right ventricle, atria are thinner. So, the left ventricle has dominance to flex the current towards it; this is normal having QRS axis +0° to +90°.

RIGHT VENTRICULAR HYPERTROPHY

Right ventricular hypertrophy is found in limited cases where both volume and pressure overload occur, as in severe COPD with pulmonary hypertension.

Limb leads:

The commonest feature of RVH is **Right axis deviation (RAD)**. So, normal QRS axis swings to right between +90° to +180°; to be sure, it must exceed +100°, i.e., in lead I (0°) must show negativity for sure.

Precordial leads:

Normal electrical dominance of left ventricle snatched by hypertrophied right ventricle, so also the 'R wave progression' (Page 15, Fig. 14) and large 'R wave' may be found at V_1 overlaying right ventricle and small 'R wave' at V_5 (R wave progression reversed). In nutshell,

- ✓ Lead V_1: R is larger than S
- ✓ Lead V_6: S in larger than R   * Rule out Dextrocardia!

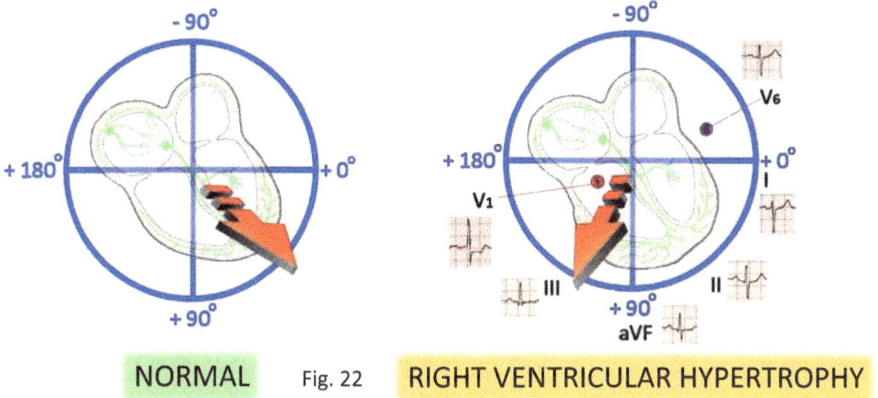

Fig. 22

LEFT VENTRICULAR HYPERTROPHY

Left ventricular muscle mass increased by exercising regularly, i.e., working against high-pressure gradient as in systemic hypertension for long time and become hypertrophied; with more mass its dominance over right ventricle increased; mean electrical vector swings leftward, ensues **left axis deviation (LAD).**

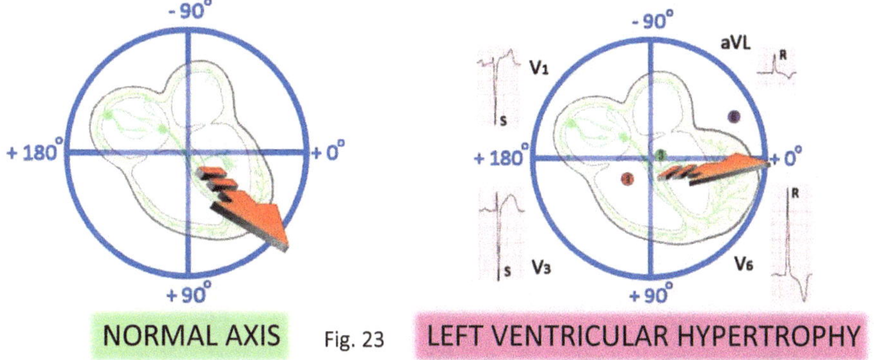

Fig. 23

Taller 'R wave' amplitude in the leads overlying the left ventricle proofs the increased dominance and hypertrophy of the structure beneath and increases 'S wave' amplitude in the leads overlying right ventricle. Precordial leads are more specific than limb leads to detect LVH.

Precordial leads criteria:

1. R wave amplitude in V_5 / V_6 + S wave amplitude in V_1 / V_2 exceeds 35 mm
2. R wave amplitude in V_5 exceeds 26 mm
3. R wave amplitude in V_6 exceeds 20 mm
4. R wave amplitude in V_5 is less than R wave amplitude in V_6

Limb leads criteria:

5. R wave amplitude in aVL exceeds 11 mm
6. R wave amplitude in I exceeds 13 mm
7. R wave amplitude in aVF exceeds 20 mm
8. R wave amplitude in I + S wave amplitude in III exceeds 25 mm
9. Most valued criteria (Cornell's) to judge the LVH is the combination of one limb and one precordial lead as, **R wave amplitude in aVL + S wave amplitude in V_3 exceeds 28 mm in men and 20 mm in women.**

Though generally criterion no. 1 is followed globally as a standard.

Try the ECG below, enquire criteria of LVH can you get and suits you:

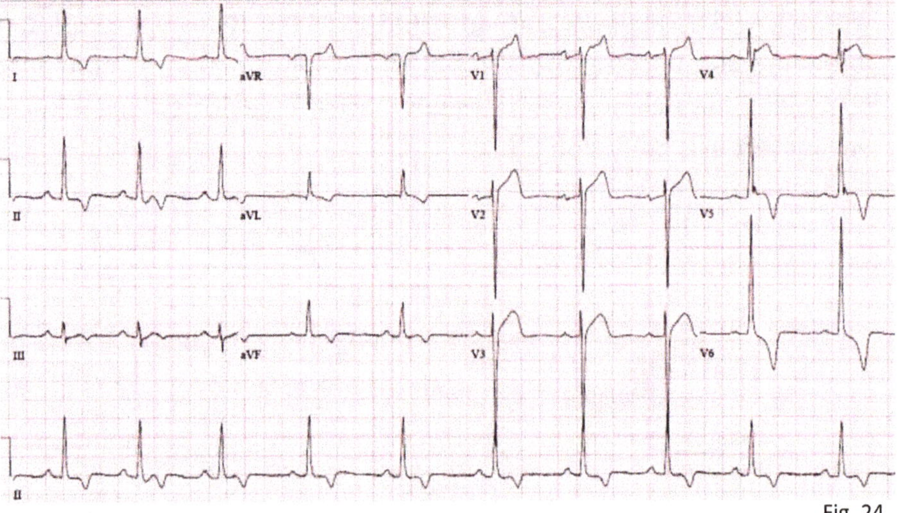

Fig. 24

What criteria do we have? Note in exercise book and recapitulate all

BI-VENTRICULAR HYPERTROPHY

The combined effect of both hypertrophied ventricle, dominant left ventricle steals all expressions of RVH. Rarely criteria of RVH in limb leads can be found as RAD and criteria of LVH in precordial leads.

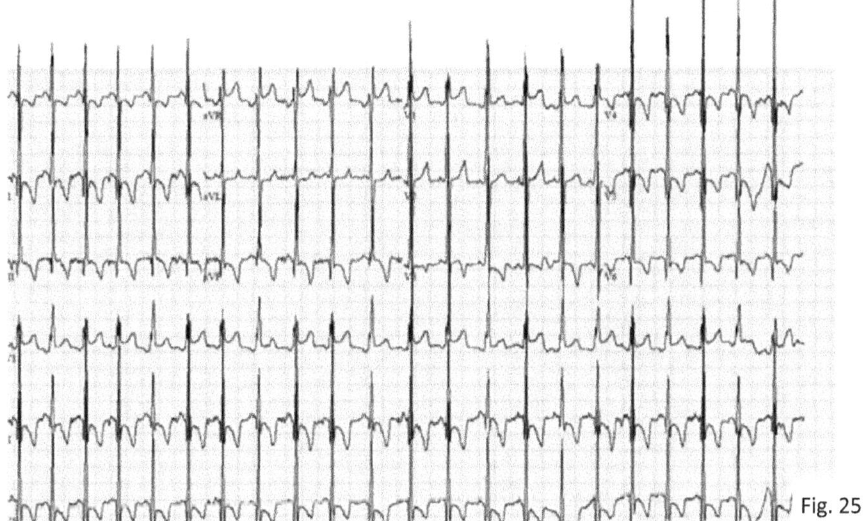

Fig. 25

VENTRICULAR HYPERTROPHY ALTERING REPOLARIZATION

ST segment plus T wave represents, end of ventricular depolarization to the end of ventricular repolarization. Ventricular hypertrophy sometimes may significantly modify the ST-T configuration, notably in severe hypertrophy; called 'secondary repolarization abnormality.'

ST depression, T wave inversion, ST & T intermingled and for single asymmetric wave where gradual downslope and abrupt upstroke seen; axis too no longer follows QRS, this change reflects on the leads which represents the area of hypertrophy so also having tall R waves.

Pediatric heart *is quite different, in the full-term baby, right and left ventricular masses are almost equal; right ventricular dominance even more than left in case of pre-terms. From the age till adolescent, left ventricular dominance increases proportionately. So, ECG of newborn or pre-term to be judged accordingly. Amplitude is also low in pre-terms, sharply rises till the age of 3-month, stable till puberty then gradually reduces as age advances.*

THIS PAGE INTENTIONALLY LEFT BLANK

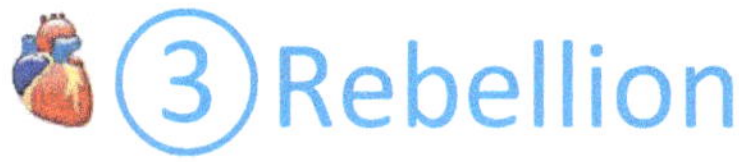 ③ Rebellion

When the administration falls, there is the beginning of 'Law of fish;' i.e., small fish become prey to bigger fish. It is heartbroken to know that the heart is no exception! If the 'Pacemaker' fails, the next big brother acts as boss and so on. In extreme conditions grand rebellion (ectopic foci) happen and there is chaos, where everyone tries to whip weaker one and vicious cycle sets in. Oh! Yes, some rebellion is lifesaving too, whether it may be sought by mother nature or a ventricular ectopic!

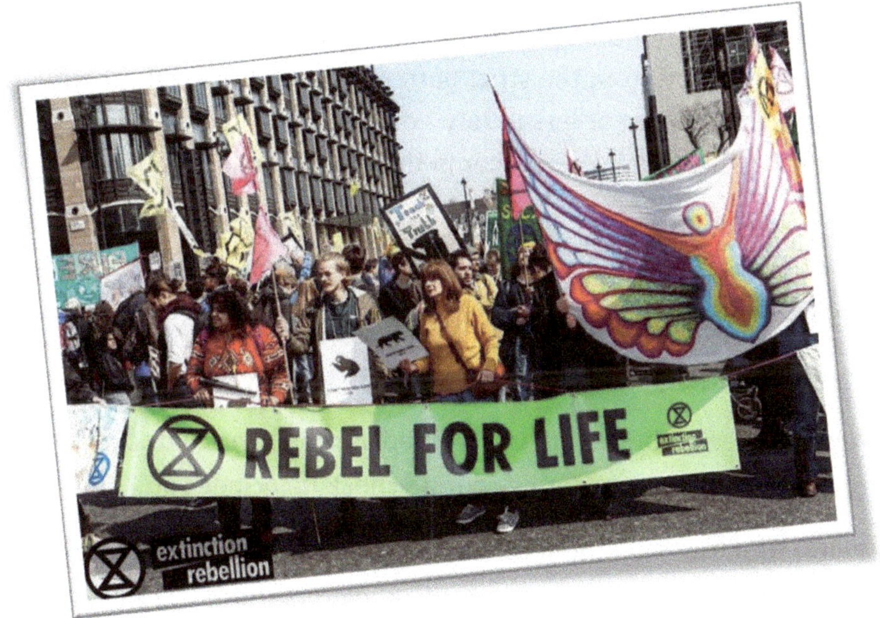

💔 Dysrhythmia

Not Arrhythmia (A=not, means no rhythm) but DYSRHYTHMIA is the correct term to mention the irregular / faulty rate and rhythm or both, of the conducting system of the heart.

➤ **NORMAL CARDIAC RHYTHM** should have:
1. HEART RATE   : 60-100 bpm
2. ORIGIN FROM   : SA node
3. TRANSMISSION   : Normal conduction pathway
4. VELOCITY   : Normal velocity

If cardiac rhythm breaks any of the above rule, called DYSRHYTHMIA.

Dysrhythmia is not always worrying, even some dysrhythmia saves life. Little derailment from the strict path is normal. As in highly competent Yogis, even 30 bpm or less is very normal; single aberrant beat derived other than SA node, often occur in the mass healthy population.

Some dysrhythmia is ominous, imminent life-threatening situation seeks immediate intervention to prevent sudden death. ECG is the best tool to determine the dysrhythmia and helps saving lives.

➤ **How to suspect a 'REBELLION' heart?**

Anyone breaks above 4 rules, stamped as rebellion. Many dysrhythmias revealed non-intently during routine checkup includes an ECG.

Palpitation is the commonest manifestation of dysrhythmia. The patient may complain of recurrent *acceleration and deceleration*; fast or slow, which may be regular or irregular; *long pause between beats*. Feeling varies from trivial to dreadful goose-bump.

Serious symptoms appear when dysrhythmia results in low cardiac output, compromising the heart's ability to pump blood effectively; *dizziness* even *syncope* ensues.

Rapid dysrhythmias seek excess oxygen demand and ensues *'angina'* when fail to accomplish demand-supply balance. Sudden onset of dysrhythmia precipitates serious hemodynamic imbalance, eventually resulting *Congestive Cardiac Failure* (CCF). Sometimes the first manifestation of dysrhythmia may be *sudden death*, which mostly noticed in the patients having Acute Myocardial Infarction (AMI).

Future 'rebel' too can be identified by the earlier changes in ECG, e.g., discovering 'prolonged QT-interval,' as seed of the fatal dysrhythmias.

💔 Background of the 'REBELLION'

Behind every REBEL, there should be factor(s), though very subtle and obscure but careful case analysis allows manageable factors to care off.

HI DR B SEN, the mnemonic may be used to remember the factors:

1. **HYPOXIA**: Lack of oxygen make myocardium to suffer – severe lung diseases, acuter pulmonary embolus, etc.
2. **IRRITABILITY, INFECTION**: Fully reversible MI without permanent damage to myocardium provokes temporary irritability. Covid-19 infection.
3. **DRUGS**: Iatrogenic, e.g., antiallergics, antacids; oddly many antiarrhythmics cause dysrhythmia!
4. **ROUSE**: Sympathetic arousal provokes dysrhythmia, e.g., Anxiety, excitement, exercise, hyperthyroidism, CCF, etc.
5. **BRADYCARDIA**: Unusually slow heart rate may precipitate dysrhythmia. E.g., sick-sinus syndrome.
6. **STRETCH**: Both hypertrophy and enlargement provoke dysrhythmia. E.g., CCF, valvular diseases.
7. **ELECTROLYTE**: Principally Potassium (K) in lack or excess provokes dysrhythmia, Calcium (Ca) and Magnesium (Mg) can also take part.
8. **NARCOTICS**: Caffeine, nicotine, and illegals, as amphetamine, cocaine, other stimulants provoke ominous dysrhythmia and sudden death.

➢ How to count the rate?

Heart rate is first to check, and quite easy to enumerate from strip. Recap, as the horizontal axis measures time: the motor rotates in such a speed that each small square corresponds to 0.04 second, and the large one (0.04 sec x 5 small squares) to 0.2 second (Page 6, Fig. 4), thus 5 large square represents 1 minute and so on.

1. Get an 'R wave' falls or almost falls at, one of the thick lines.
2. Count the number of large squares (L) until the next 'R wave.'
3. If the next 'R wave' does not fall at thick line, count small squares (s) to get it.
4. Now, the Heart rate = $\dfrac{1500}{(L\times5)+s}$ beat per minute (bpm).

Let us try the Heart rate of the ECG given below:

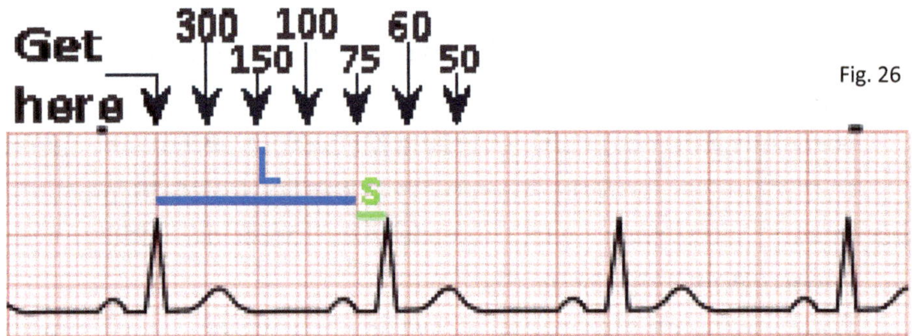

What do we get? Here 'L = 4' and 's=3. So,

Heart rate = $\dfrac{1500}{(4\times5)+3}$ = $\dfrac{1500}{23}$ = 65 bpm (approx.).

Another method:

Every ECG strip is marked at 3 second intervals (every 15th large square). Count the number of cycles between two such markings (i.e., 6 seconds apart) and multiply by 10 and get heart rate.

💔 'REBELLIONS' do five basic types of breach –

1. Breaks speed rules only – Follow the usual pathway but either *slow* (bradyarrhythmia/bradycardia) *or fast* (tachyarrhythmia/tachycardia).
2. Originates from normal site and follows usual pathway but encounters unfortunate – *delay and even blocks.*
3. Originates other than (ectopic) or added to normal 'pacemaker (SA node)' – *ectopic rhythms.*
4. Keep in loops – *reentrant tachyarrhythmia.*
5. Nothing is right with them; follows accessory shortcut pathway, bypassing the normal – *preexcitation.*

♥ Originating from SA node

Normal pacemaker of heart is SA node where depolarization spontaneously originates and propagates at a rate 60-100 bpm.

<u>Sinus Arrhythmia:</u> In some individuals often, ECG reveals slightly regular irregular rhythm. It is the change of heart rate with respiration. During inspiration, vagal output decreases and heart rate increases and during expiration heart rate decreased. It is very normal.

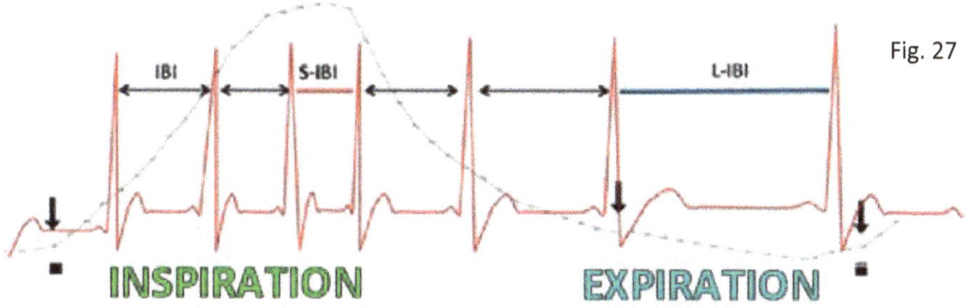

<u>Sinus Bradycardia:</u> When the heart rate decreases below 60 bpm, called bradycardia. In some non-pathological conditions too, sinus bradycardia may be present, e.g., in trained yogis and athletes due to increased vagal tone etc. It is found in hypometabolic state early stage of acute MI, medications such as Calcium-channel-blockers, beta-blockers, etc.

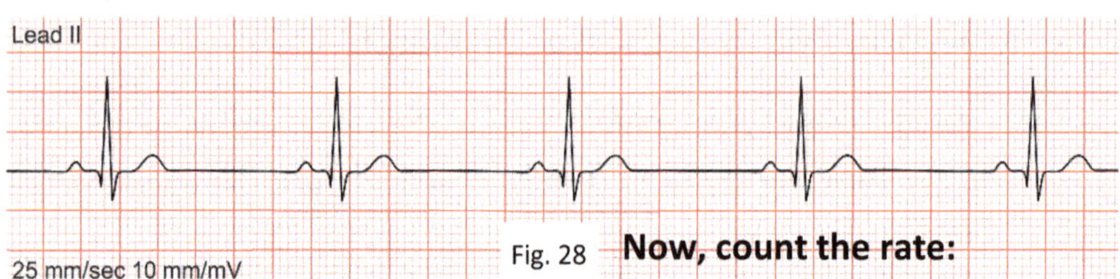

<u>Sinus Tachycardia:</u> When the heart rate increases above 100 bpm, called tachycardia. In some non-pathological conditions too, as during pregnancy, strenuous exercise, etc. It is found during fever, hypermetabolic state, severe pulmonary disease, CCF, Ehler DS, etc.

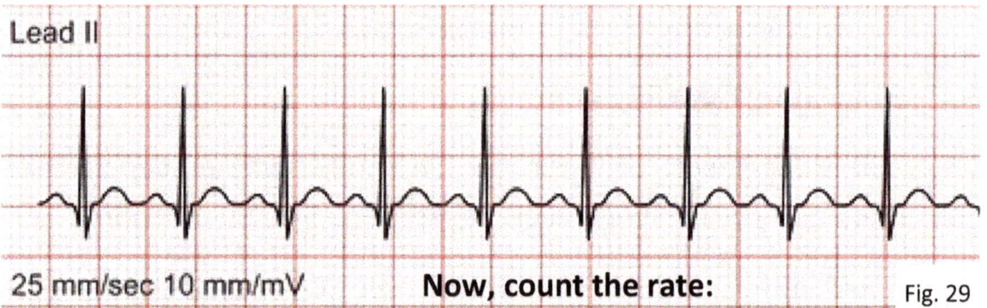

<u>Relative Bradycardia:</u> Fever proportionally increases heart rate, but in some fevers, heart rate is slower than expected, e.g., typhoid, dengue.

<u>Sinus Arrest:</u> SA node stopped generation or SA node generates but there is an 'exit block;' in both situations ECG will not show any electrical activity and show flat line. Prolonged sinus inactivity is called 'asystole.' It is near impossible* to detect whether the electrical inactivity is due to sinus arrest or failure to propagate.

* With sinus arrest, firing of the SA node occur at any random time BUT with 'exit block' as the SA node is firing silently, when block is removed, the SA node resumes depolarizing after a pause which is exact numeral multiple of the normal cycle (1 or 2 missed P wave).

<u>Escape Beat:</u> All myocardial cells have potential to act as pacemaker; on sinus arrest the next fastest pacemaker takes charge and generate 'rescue beat' which is other than (non-sinus) the SA node called '**escape beat**' to save life. Some rebels are lifesaving! In below ECG, see the long pause, 5th beat restoring electrical activity having no P wave.

Fig. 30

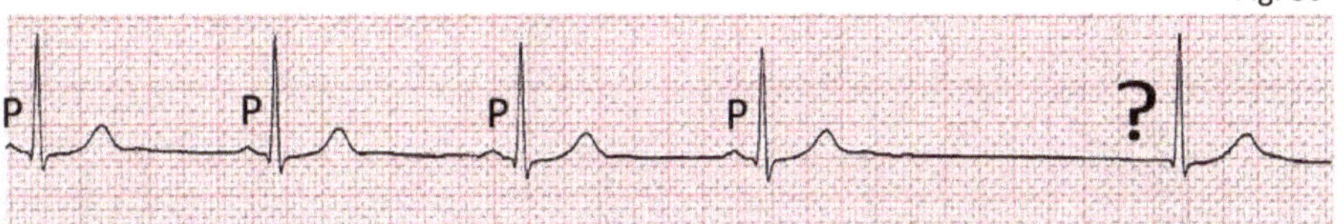

Non-sinus pacemakers have their own intrinsic rate. *Atrial pacemaker* fires at 60-75 bpm; *junctional pacemaker* (pacemaker cells near AV node) fires at 40-60 bpm; *ventricular pacemaker* fires at 30-45 bpm. Anyone of these can rescue the sinus arrest generating only one or, on need, series of escape beats. Junctional escape is the commonest.

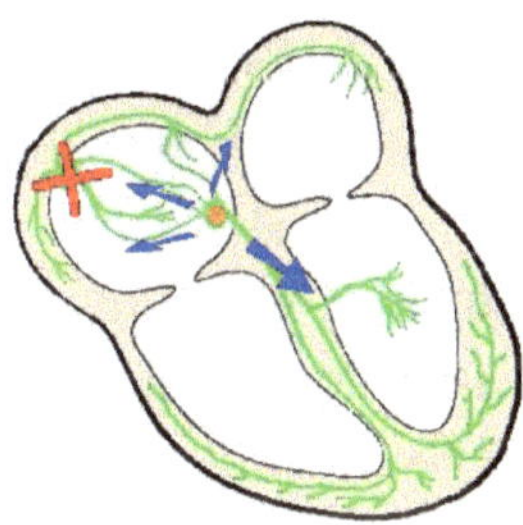

Fig. 31

In junctional escape, depolarization starts near the AV node; so, atrial depolarization occurs in abnormal way and thus no or abnormal P wave. Sometimes, a 'retrograde P wave' may be found with 180° reversal of mean axis of P wave, which proves that the depolarization wave is moving backward from junctional region to atria.

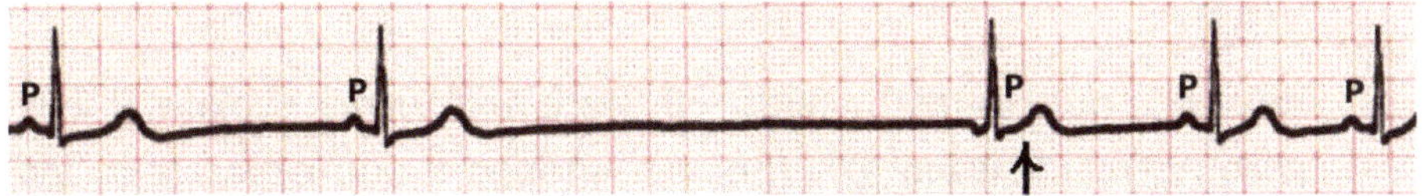

Non-sinus dysrhythmia occurs in two ways, - **ectopic** and **re-entry**. *Ectopic rhythm* is that one which originates other than SA node due to the increased automaticity at the cellular level; there may be a single focus or a wandering one. Until this ectopic focus cannot overdrive the rate of performing pacemaker, heart beats under the whip of that pacemaker. So, only when the ectopic focus firing at higher rate, became electrically significant enough and expressed in ECG.

Re-entry is the problem in wave transmission. It is quite easy to understand. Assume, a wave of depolarization arriving at two adjacent regions as path Fast (F) & Slow (S) of the myocardium.

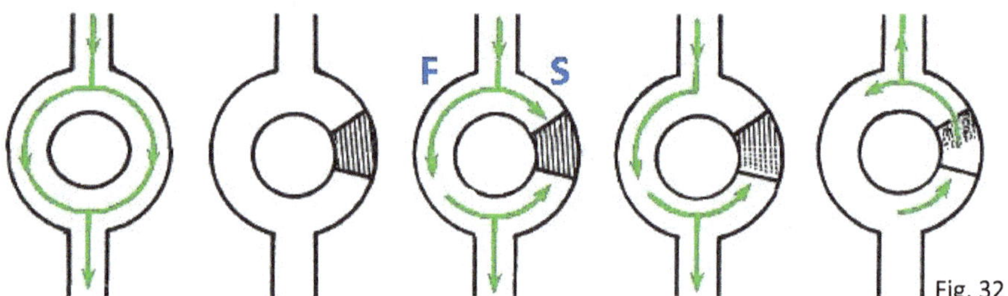

Fig. 32

In the left most picture, the wave conducted through path F & S with same rate and progress further reunited and untroubled.

In other pictures, there is a block in path-S, so, the wave conducted through path-S delayed (due to Ischemic, fibrotic, etc. changes) than path-F. Depolarization wave come out from path-F is earlier and can wind back towards path-S and if found refractory, starts an endless electrical loop (re-entry) circuit along the two pathways and send impulses to all directions.

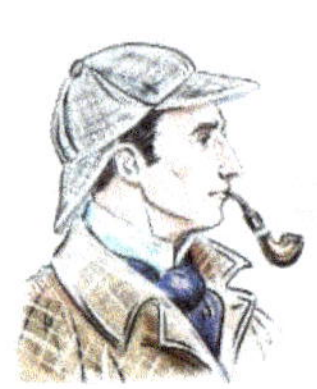

Re-entry loop(s) differ widely, it may be confined to a single small loop or may loop through whole of any chamber of heart.

The SIGN OF FOUR

1. Presence of normal P waves – If there are normal looking P waves with normal P wave axis (positive in lead II and negative in aVR), then the origin of dysrhythmia is almost surely within the atria. If P waves are absent, then the rhythm originated below atria.

    The presence of P wave with abnormal P wave axis indicates,

(a) Atria activated from focus deriving from atria except SA node, or

(b) Retrograde activation from a site within AV node or ventricles, i.e., wave flowing backwards to atria through AV or through any other accessory pathway connecting atria and ventricle.

2. QRS-complex duration – if <0.12 seconds, the depolarization conducting through normal pathway which indicates that, the focus is at or above the AV node i.e., supraventricular in origin and wider QRS-complex indicates ventricular origin typically.
3. Relationship between P wave & QRS-complex – if both go 'made for each other' way, single P wave go before each QRS-complex, then the focus is almost surely of SA nodal or atrial origin. We also can notice divorce, where atria and ventricle depolarize independently scribing complete discordance between P wave & QRS-complex named as **AV dissociation** and like all divorce between parents, child (cardiac output) suffer the most!
4. Regularity of rhythm – Regularity or irregularity is instantly recognizable attributes of a particular dysrhythmia and occasionally very crucial.

💔 SUPRAVENTRICULAR DYSRHYTHMIA

In the heart, there is a moderator between atria and ventricles, the AV node; and we know that our main concern is with cardiac output concern with ventricular contraction following electrical stimulus. So, for practical purposes, we can divide dysrhythmia into 'supraventricular' and 'ventricular' in origin.

Supraventricular dysrhythmias, derive in atria and AV node.

Atrial and Junctional Premature Beats

Single ectopic supraventricular beat originating in the atria is called atrial premature beat; resulting Premature Atrial Contraction or PAC & those originating from the vicinity of the AV node is called Junctional premature beat. These are usual phenomena, found in normal hearts but can initiate continuous dysrhythmia.

Atrial premature beat scribes in ECG as changes in P wave timing and contour as follows:

Timing: An atrial premature beat comes too early and scribes in ECG earlier than the next anticipated normal sinus beat.

Contour: Changing of usual pathway of wave propagation occurs if site of the ectopic is distant from SA node and results change in P wave axis.

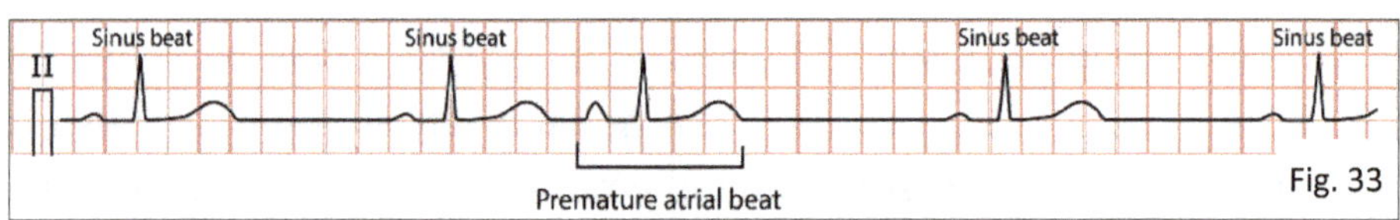

Fig. 33

In junctional premature beats, usually no visible P wave; sometimes rather, there may be retrograde P wave, like the junctional escape beats seen with sinus arrest as a rescue phenomenon. It is difficult to differentiate by ECG, but 'Junctional Premature Beat' occurs EARLY (hence the term), and 'Escape beat' occurs LATE (as a rescue).

Fig. 34

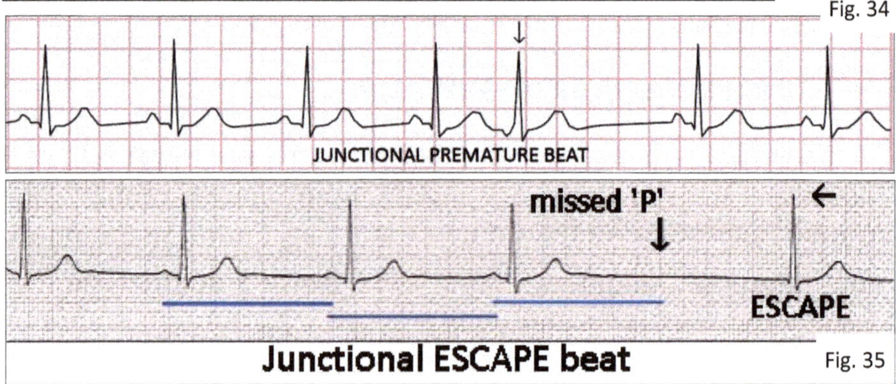

Fig. 35

As both conveyed via normal pathway through ventricles, QRS wave scribes normal timing so as usual narrow complex.

Continuous supraventricular dysrhythmia are diverse types:

1. AV Nodal Reentrant Tachycardia (AVNRT), also known as Paroxysmal Supraventricular Tachycardia (PSVT)
2. Atrial **Flutter (AF)**
3. Atrial **fibrillation (Af)**
4. Multifocal Atrial Tachyarrhythmia (MAT)
5. Paroxysmal Atrial Tachyarrhythmia (PAT)/Ectopic Atrial Tachycardia
6. AV Reciprocating Tachyarrhythmia (AVRT)

💔 AV NODAL REENTRANT TACHYCARDIA (AVNRT)

It is usually benign, regular, and the most common type found even in the persons with perfect heart. Sudden start and sudden go, initiated by a Premature Supraventricular beat (so PSVT); usually found in guys from party having nexus of coffee, alcohol, absolute excitement and complaints of palpitation, shortness of breath, dizziness, and even syncopal attack. Heart rate remains between 150-250 bpm, which is usually led by a re-entry path circling within the AV node. *Retrograde P waves* may be present in leads II and III but confirmatory is having pseudo-R' in lead V_1. P waves often buried in QRS are so unidentifiable.

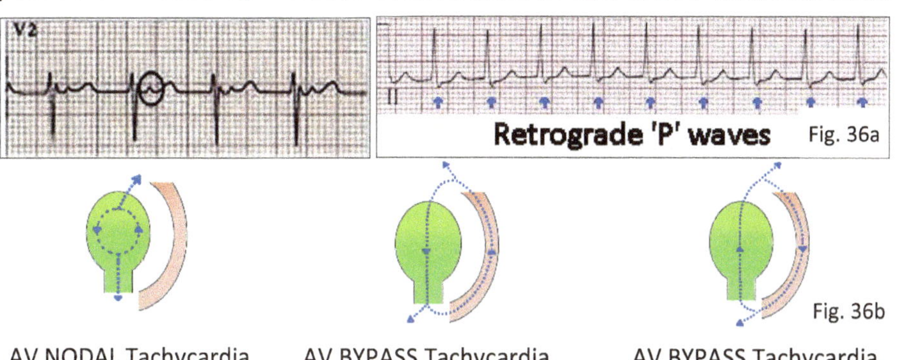

| AV NODAL Tachycardia | AV BYPASS Tachycardia (Orthodromic) | AV BYPASS Tachycardia (Antidromic) |

💔 **Lifesaving Carotid Massage** – I lost my father at his 75 years, who did not get this assistance sadly, when got (?) arrhythmic attack on hurry to catch the train, having known paroxysmal atrial fibrillation (PA**f**), uncontrolled DM-II, cardiomyopathy, on cephalosporin for suspected UTI and recent fall which possibly provoked Hypotension, A**f** and cardiac arrest (see also – Kounis syndrome – Chapter 7).

Carotid massage used both diagnostic and treatment purposes; near the common carotid bifurcation, baroreceptors present, which senses the changes in blood pressure. Gentle pressure on *single carotid* (just enough to dip a tennis ball) near mandibular angle on right or left side by reflex slows down heart rate by stimulating Vagus nerve; depressing SA node and slows down AV node conduction on left side, respectively.

❤️ ATRIAL FLUTTER (AF)

Atrial **F**lutter usually happens in diseased heart, it is regular but faster than AVNRT. P wave rate 250-350 bpm usually arises out of single endless reentrant pathway around the annulus of the tricuspid valve. Due to faster rate baseline is absent and 'saw-tooth' scribed on ECG. AV-node being slow, thus refractory most of the time; can't pass all stimuli and produce AV-block. 2:1 block is commonest, which may be 3:1 or even 4:1 block. Note, as carotid massage increase the block; a 2:1 AV block may lead to 3:1 or 4:1 block. Aslo note, as Atrial Flutter originates above the AV-node it can't break the dysrhythmia.

Fig. 37

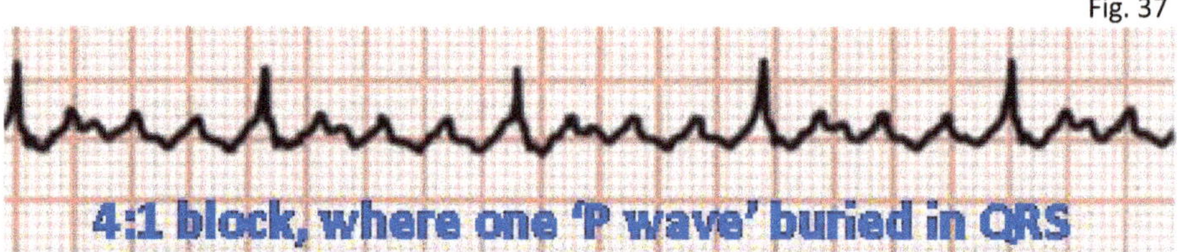

P wave axis in flutter waves differs upon whether the reentrant current around tricuspid valve rotates clockwise scribing positive sawtooth or if counter-clockwise, scribing negative sawtooth pattern.

❤️ ATRIAL fibrillation (Af)

Atrial activity fully disorganized, several minute reentrant pathways are the sole offender, more than 500 bpm approach to the AV node without any pattern. So, **no 'P wave'** found, which is replaced by little **undulating fibrillation (f) wave or flat baseline**. AV node being perplexed, allows impulses down towards ventricles now and then, scribes **irregularly irregular QRS complex** rated **> 150 bpm**.

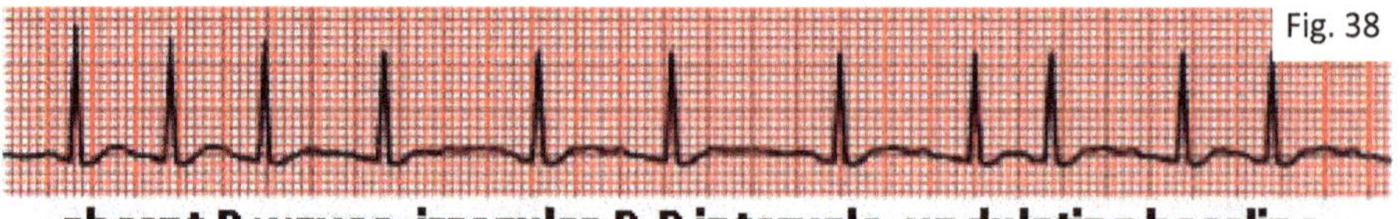
Fig. 38

absent P waves, irregular R-R intervals, undulating baseline

❤ MULTIFOCAL ATRIAL TACHYARRHYTHMIA (MAT)

It is an irregular rhythm of 100 – 200 bpm; as the name suggest, due to random firing from different ectopic atrial sites, usually found in the patients with severe lung diseases. MAT can be distinguished from atrial fibrillation by the easily identifiable 'P' wave prior to each 'QRS'. As in MAT, foci are changing so there are changes to P wave (at least three different morphologies) and PR interval. Carotid massage have no effect on MAT, thus used as clinical tool for differentiation.

Sometimes the rate may be lower than 100 bpm (so not a tachycardia) and thus called 'Wandering Atrial Pacemaker'; as MAT here too, three different 'P' wave morphologies present but there will be at least two beats of each 'P' wave morphology before the pacemaker moves to the other site and scribes changed morphology of 'P' and PR interval.

❤ PAROXYSMAL ATRIAL TACHYARRHYTHMIA (PAT)

It is a **regular** rhythm rating 100-200 bpm, either due to higher automaticity of an ectopic atrial focus (common) or due to re-entry phenomenon within atria. Now, automatic type shows a *gradual speed-up at start and slow-down at end.* On contrary, re-type starts *abrupt* with an atrial premature beat, also known as **atypical atrial flutter.**

PAT and AVNRT are very difficult to differentiate and at times impossible. Only if there is gradual speed-up and slow-down, is possible to be PAT. In addition carotid massage will slow or cease AVNRT but almost uneffected on PAT.

Fig. 39

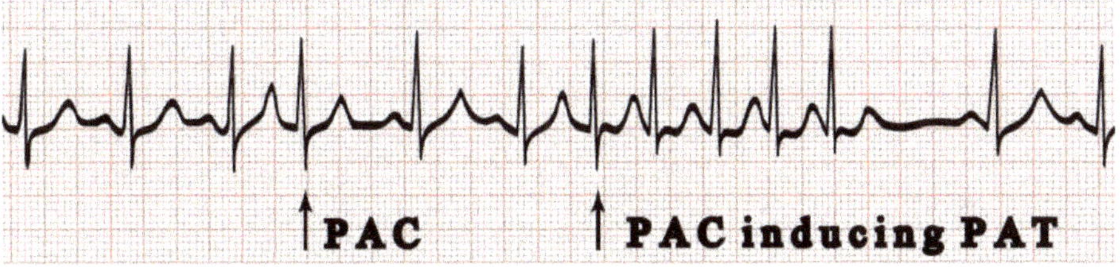

 **SICK-SINUS SYNDROME (TACHY-BRADY SYNDROME)**

It is the alternate episode of supraventricular tachycardia as Atrial fibrillation, alters with bradycardia.; which indicates major esoteric issue to the conducting system. Usually caused by mutation of myocardial sodium channels and often associated with myopia!

<u>NOTE</u>

💔 VENTRICULAR DYSRHYTHMIA

These are the rhythm disorders creating below AV node.

PREMATURE VENTRICULAR CONTRACTION (PVC)

It is the commonest ventricular dysrhythmia. As we know any rhythm that takes unusual pathway takes longer time and bizarre, here is also no exception, **QRS complex is wide and bizarre in PVCs**. Though QRS may not appear wide in all leads (shorter/normal to the leads near focus); the QRS duration should be ≥ 0.12 seconds in most leads.

PVCs usually followed by prolonged compensatory pause before the next beat scribes. Sometimes, between two normally conducted beats, PVC occur without compensatory pause – **interpolated PVCs**. Rarely retrograde 'P' waves also can be seen.

💔 Isolated PVCs also sometimes scribe in absolutely normal hearts BUT if found with AMI is dangerous, which can trigger life threatening arrythmias – Vtach or Ventricular fibrillation.

PVCs are usually innocent till it contributes less than 10% of the beats, else it may ensue remodelling of the myocardium by developing dilated cardiomyopathy; sometimes it also precipitates ventricular tachycardia, ventricular fibrillation and even death. These are the 'rules of malignancy' in nut-shell:

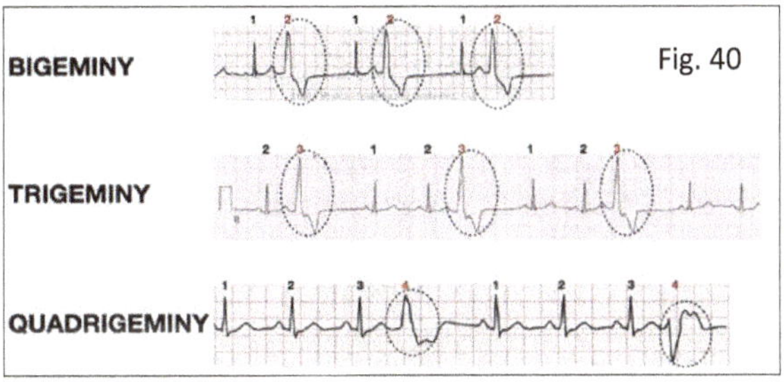

BIGEMINY	Fig. 40
TRIGEMINY	
QUADRIGEMINY	

RIGHT vs LEFT PVC

The ventricle from which the PVC originates best recognized by V_1. If PVC is mostly positive in V_1, means depolarization anteriorly rightwords, so originates at posteriorly located LV (c.f. IHD) ; on contrary, if predominantly negative in V_1, means depolariztion posteriorly leftward, so originates at anteriorly located RV.

1. PVCs more than 10%.
2. Consecutive PVCs, especially more than two in a row.
3. PVCs of different morphology.
4. PVCs falling over previous T wave; i.e., 'R on T' phenomenon. Repolarization is very crucial to cardiac cycle and PVC fall during repolarization may trigger ventricular tachycardia.
5. PVC occuring in the setting of an AMI.

However, controlling these malignance PVCs, practically have no beneficial outcome to reduce mortality.

💔 VENTRICULAR TACHYCARDIA

It is nothing but the three or more PVCs in row rated at 120-200 bpm. Vtach lasting more than 30 seconds or associated with hemodynamic instability, requires immediate intervention else cardiac arrest.

Morphology of the Vtach is usually uniform, unless provoked following acute ischemia, MI, conditions causing prolongation of QT interval; e.g., antifungal; antihistaminic; antibiotics like erythromycin, azithromycin; antiarrhythmics; antidepressants; massive electrolyte imbalance (hypocalcemia/hypokalemia/etc.); etc.

All of these lengthens ventricular repolarization (T wave) and PVCs get enough space to fall on T, which eventually initiates 'torsade de pointes' (twisting of the points). It looks like ordinary Vtach but QRS are spiral around the baseline changing axes and amplitudes beat to beat.

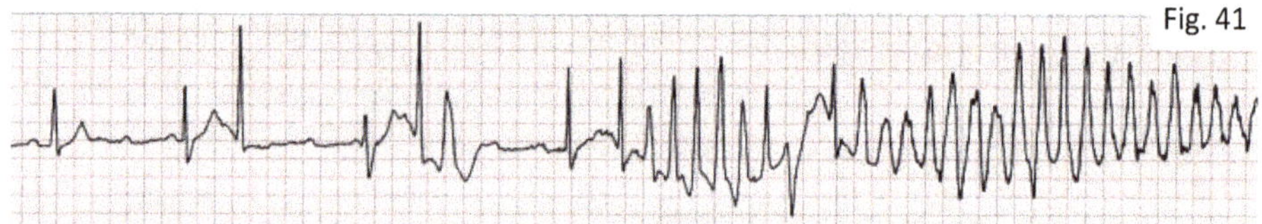

Fig. 41

💔 VENTRICULAR FIBRILLATION (V-fib)

This ominous condition is the commonest deadly arrhythmia of adults, lead to sudden cardiac arrest, accounts almost 50% of all cardiac deaths. As in this state there is no cardiac output being just a quivering mass, CPR and defibrillator to be used immediately to rescue the patient.

They are two types,

a) Coarse ventricular fibrillation – Tall peaks and deep vallies.
b) Fine ventricular fibrillation – Short peaks and shallow vallies.

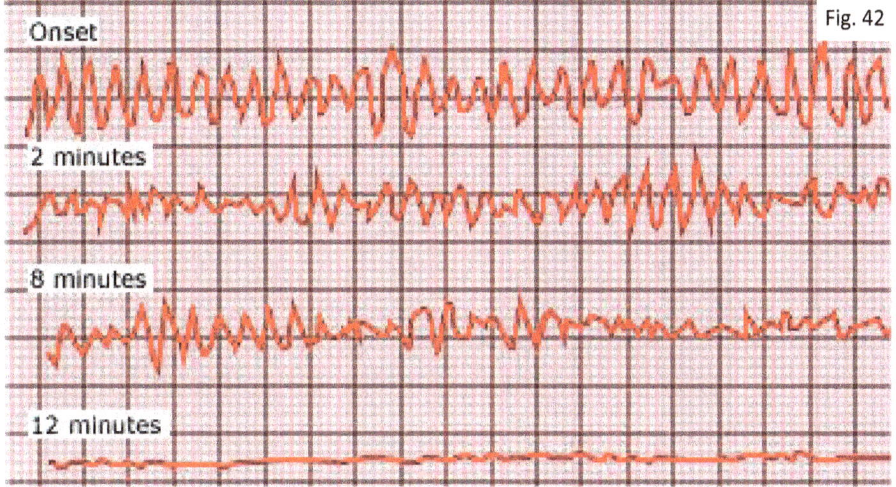

Continuous ECG strip: At the onset of ventricular fibrillation, QRS complexes are regular but widened, and of tall amplitude; indicating a more organized ventricular tachyarrhythmia. Later, the rhythm becomes more disorganized with higher amplitude fibrillatory waves; this is coarse VF. After a longer period, the fibrillatory waves become fine VF and climaxing in asystole.

💔 Refractory V-fib: When ventricular fibrillation continues even after three successive shocks from a defibrillator – called refractory V-fib.

💔 IDIOVENTRICULAR RHYTHM

It is very similar to ventricular tachycardia, except the rate < 60 bpm (Fig. 43), which alternately called "slow ventricular tachycardia"! When the rate accelerated to 50-100 bpm, called "_accelerated idioventricular rhythm_" (Fig. 44). It is found occasionally during early hours after reperfusion or in birth; represents 'ventricular escape' generated to run the heart sufficiently, self limiting and rarely require any treatment.

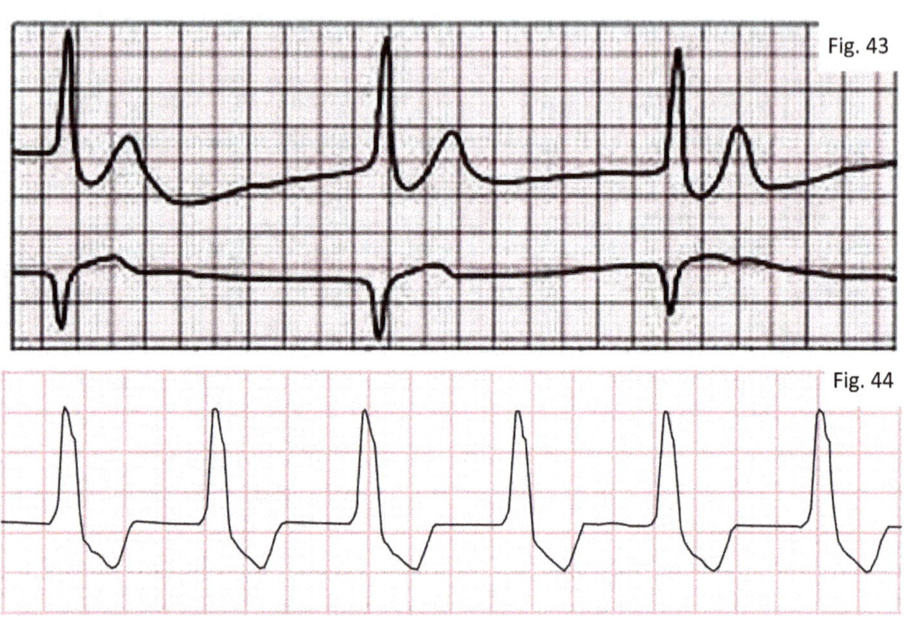

Fig. 43

Fig. 44

💔 SUPRAVENTRICULAR vs VENTRICULAR ARRHYTHMIA

It is worth mentioning that, optimum cardiac output is the sole moto of the heart pump, which directly depends upon the ventricular function rather than atrial. So, arrhythmia of the ventricle have more fatal prognosis and thus the treatment protocol have gulf of differences.

Supraventricular arrhythmia scribes 'narrow QRS' while ventricular arrhythmia scribes 'wide QRS' except in **aberrancy**; which is indistinguishable from PVC when an atrial premature beat (PAC) arises too early in the next cycle, that the Purkinje fibres in the ventricles yet not repolarized fully to catch the next one, especilly RBB being more lethargic, so still refractory → current goes down along LBB → ventricles as a whole take longer time to depolarize → broad bizarre QRS like PVC.

It is almost impossible to distinguish between them but the clues are:

In single PAC, there is a 'P' preceds the wide 'QRS' but no preceding 'P' in PVC. But in long continued arrhythmia it become harder; as both AVNRT and V-tach have same rates too.

Other clues are,

1. **A**xis: Northwest (-90 to -180 degrees), is highly specific for VT (90%)
2. **B**road complexes: Use a cut-off of > 200ms, which has a specificity of 85-90% for VT. Below this, there is too much overlap between VT and SVT with aberrancy.

    Note – variants such as Right Ventricular Outflow Tract (RVOT) VT may exhibit shorter QRS durations – as such, a narrower QRS does not exclude VT.
3. **C**oncordance: If QRS complex resemble any aberration? – if so, probably SVT else VT / antedromic AVRT.
4. **D**issociation: Any evidence of AV-dissociation is highly specific for VT.

    - P and QRS complexes at different rates.
    - **Capture beats**: where SA node transiently "captures" the ventricles, producing an isolated normal QRS complex.
    - **Fusion beats**: Occur when a sinus and ventricular beat coincide to produce a hybrid complex.
5. **E**arly part of QRS: fast / slow? - SVT with aberrancy and VT differ in the way that they engage the His-Purkinje network:

    - VT propagates from ventricular muscle, with initial slow myocyte-to-myocyte conduction time. This causes a delayed/slurred initial QRS.
    - SVT with aberrancy displays initial sharp QRS deflections that arise from the preserved bundle branch.
6. V-tach usually result of a diseased heart (post MI, CCF, etc.).
7. Carotid massage may terminate AVNRT.
8. Cannon A waves at Jugular veins in V-tach (as 75% associated with AV dissociation – no relation between 'P' an 'QRS').
9. In AVNRT – sometimes retrograde 'P' with positive deflection in lead aVR and negative deflection in lead II.
10. In AVNRT though aberrancy being supraventricular, initial deflection of QRS usually in same direction of normal QRS.

To be sure, electrophysiologic study (EPS) is the only bay, which is an invasive technique using intracardiac electrodes and source of arrhythmia can be accurately mapped.

♥ Ashman phenomenon:

Fisch criteria for the diagnosis of Ashman phenomenon –

1. Relatively long cycle immediately preceding the cycle terminated by the aberrant QRS complex
2. RBBB form aberrancy with normal orientation of the initial QRS vector, a series of wide QRS supraventricular beats is possible
3. Irregular coupling of aberrant QRS complexes
4. A short-long-short RR interval is even more likely to initiate aberration; and
5. Lack of fully compensatory pause

The refractory period of His-Purkinje system is proportionate to RR interval of the preceding beat. So, when two beats are separated by a long RR interval, the later refractory period will be relatively long.

If a premature supraventricular stimulus (short RR interval) follows a long RR interval whilst His-Purkinje system is still refractory, then the conducted beat will appear abnormal. As the refractory period of the right bundle is slightly longer than the left, the aberrantly conducted beat typically demonstrates a right bundle branch (RBBB) morphology.

Atrial fibrillation with its varying, irregular conduction, causing long and short pauses between QRS complexes, is the perfect substrate of the Ashman phenomenon.

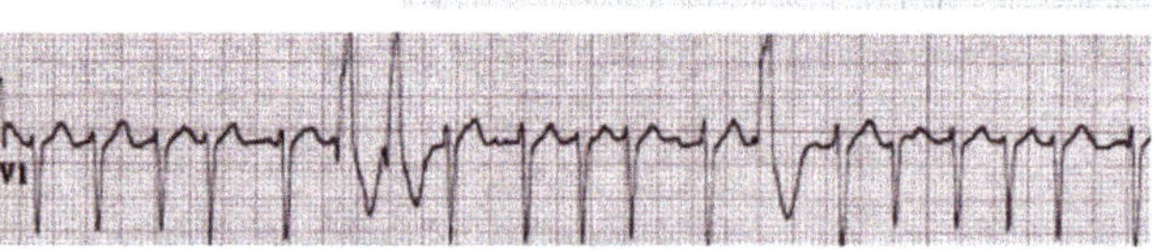

Rapid Afib with Ashman beats (long-short-wide beat sequences)	

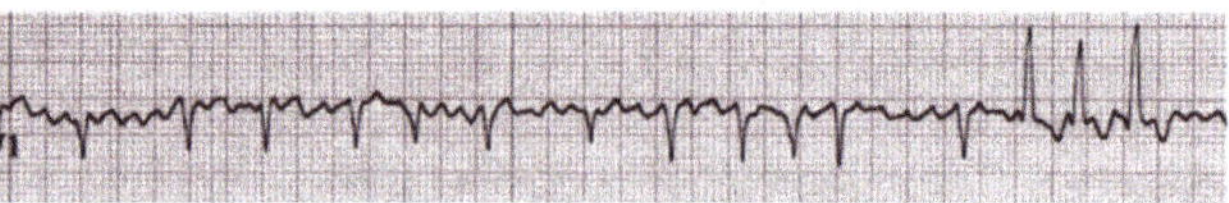

| Rapid Afib with 3 - beats run of wide beats, an example of Ashman sequences | |

Fig. 45

📍④ Network interruption

In this age, info is the prime, if not the omnipotent determinant of the force of action in any workfield; which needs uninterrupted conduction of 'current' of info through the fastest network available.

If interrupted for a while, total system failure in every field whether it is a meticulous neurosurgery / road signalling / landing a research vehicle to any celestial body to share market.

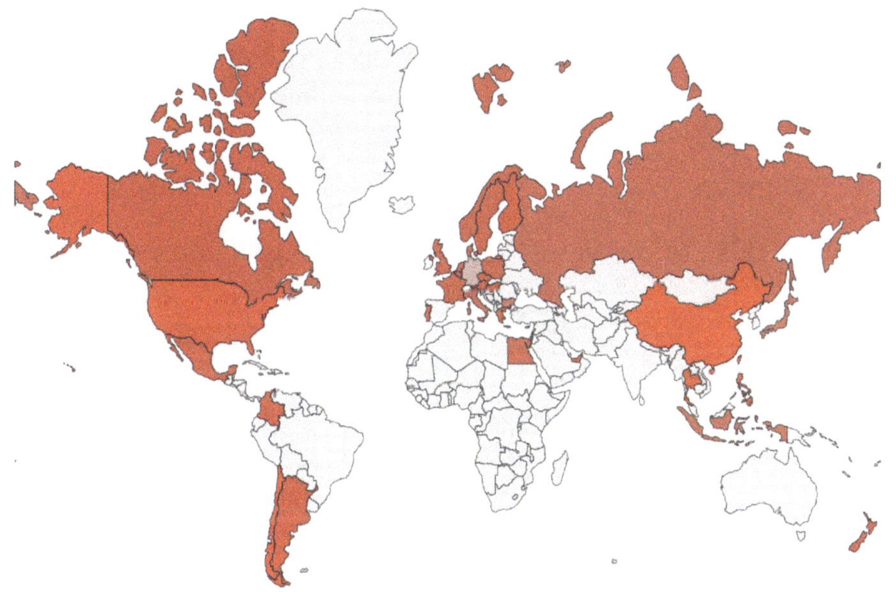

Internet outage trends during Covid-19 pandemic

The 'current' generated at SA node is of no exception. It finds the shortest and fastest way to be conducted through the whole heart. If interrupted, delay to complete jeopardise occur.

So, conduction block is, any type of obstruction or delay of the flow of 'current' along the normal conduction pathway.

Conductions blocks are classified according the anatomical location:

1. Sinus node block = 'Sinus exit block' (see page 32).
2. AV block – Any block between SA node and terminal Purkinje fibres including bundle of His.
3. Bundle Branch Block – Conduction block of right or left bundle or both; any fascicle of the left also may be blocked and termed as 'fascicular block' or 'hemiblock'.

❤️ AV – BLOCK

1° AV BLOCK: With every 'P' there is a 'QRS' but **PR interval > 0.2* sec.**

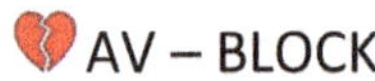
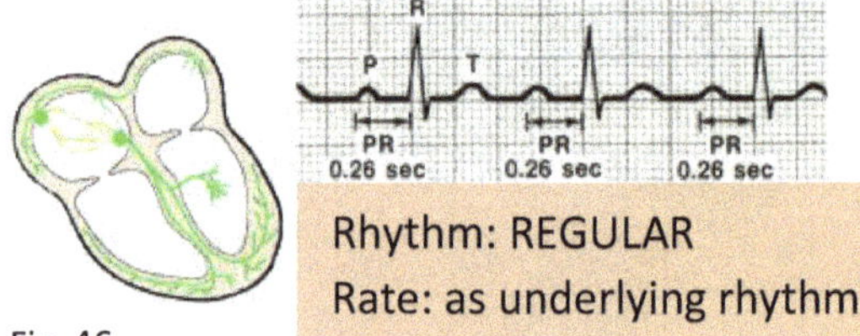

Fig. 46

Rhythm: REGULAR
Rate: as underlying rhythm
QRS: Usually, normal

Normal PR interval*

1. CHILDHOOD: 0.10-0.12
2. ADOLESCENCE: 0.12-0.16
3. ADULTHOOD: 0.14 - 0.21

2° HEART BLOCK – Mobitz type-I :
- Every 'P' not always followed by 'QRS'.
- **Progressive lengthening of PR interval**, then a 'P' is not followed by 'QRS; then recycles.

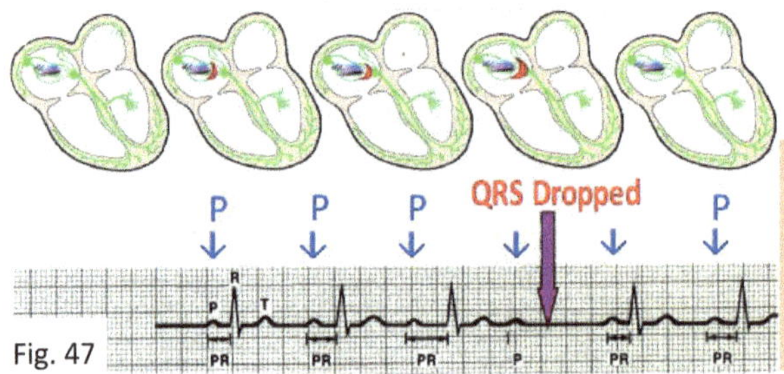

Fig. 47

Atrial rhythm: REGULAR
Ventricular rhythm: REGULAR / IRREGULAR
QRS: Normal

2° HEART BLOCK – Mobitz type-II :

- Every 'P' not always followed by 'QRS'.
- PR interval stable (normal or prolonged). Some 'P' is not followed by 'QRS' as drop beat.

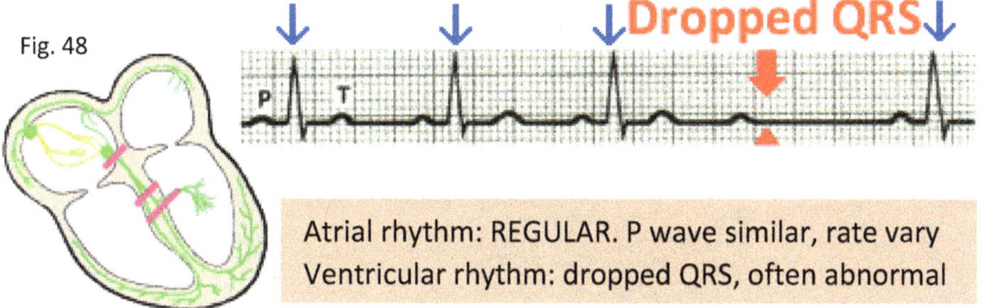

Fig. 48

RHYTHMIC (FIXED-RATIO) 2° HEART BLOCK :

- Every 'P' not always followed by 'QRS'.
- PR interval stable (normal or prolonged). Some 'P' is not followed by 'QRS' as drop beat; in a rhythm. e.g. 'QRS' after every 2nd (2:1) / 3rd (3:1) block. > 3:1 block also termed as high degree AV block

2:1 Block

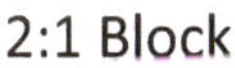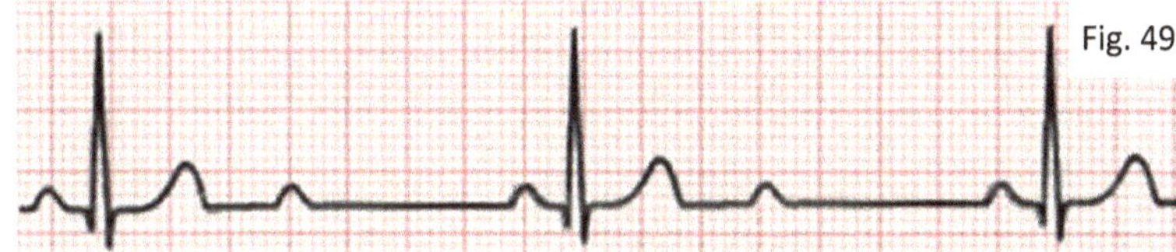

Fig. 49

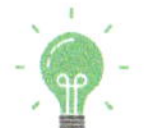WoW! : 5th heart sound!! – 5th sound is evident as added wave of the anterior mitral leaflet (G, g1) when there is slow heart rate, 2:1 block.

3:1 Block

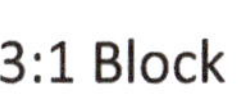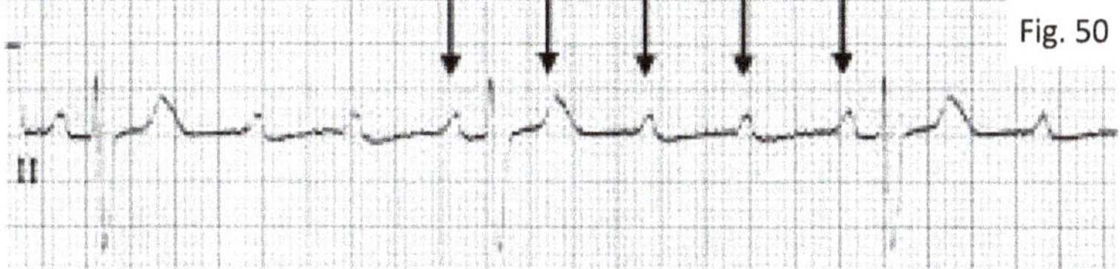

Fig. 50

COMPLETE / 3° HEART BLOCK : Complete **dissociation** between atria & ventricles. Both depolarize individually at their own rate.

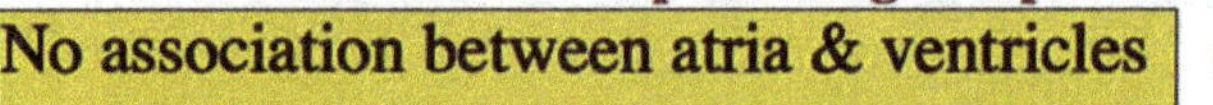

Fig. 51

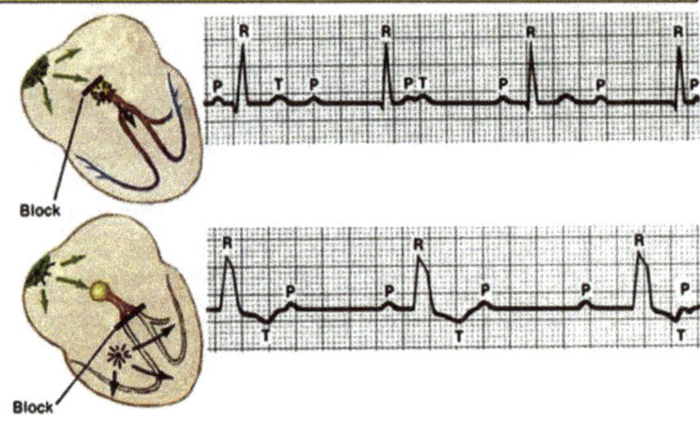

The Heart Block Poem

- If the R is far from the P, then you have a 1ˢᵗ Degree

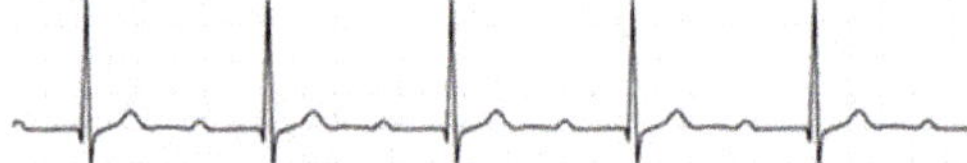

- PR gets longer, longer, longer, drop, it's a case of Wenckebach!

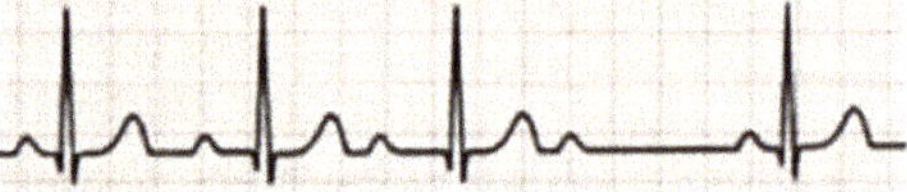

- If some R's don't get through, prepare to pace that Mobitz II!

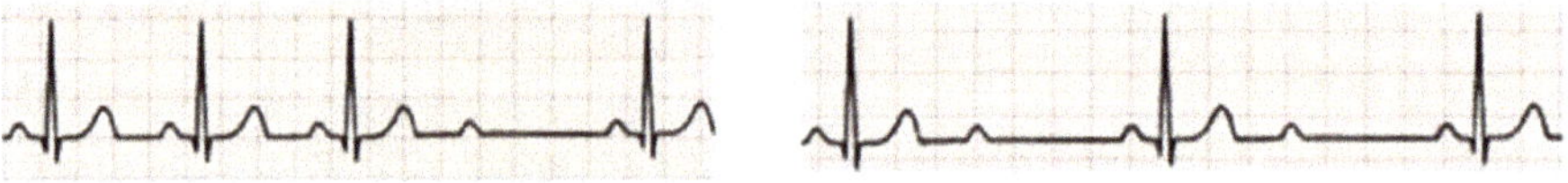

- If the R's & P's don't agree, prepare to PACE that 3ʳᵈ degree!

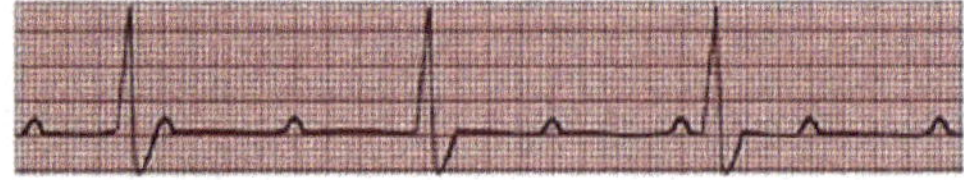

Fig. 52

💔 BUNDLE BRANCH BLOCK

This is the conduction block in left or right bundle branches.

Bundle branch block is diagnosed by looking at the breadth and shape of the QRS complex.

NORMAL	RBBB

Depolarization goes to left then right fascicles as refractory period of right fascicle is more → Ventricular septal activation responsible for the generation of 'q.' V_5 V_6 being the lateral leads and as the current goes away from V_5 V_6 towards V_1 V_2; 'q' which indicates septal activation shown in V_5 V_6 normally.

Normal activation of Left heart **but delayed conduction to Right heart** → both depolarization and repolarization affected.

Due to delayed depolarization of Right ventricle → RSR' (rSR) pattern in V_1 V_2 – 'RABBIT EAR' appearance; in V_5 V_6 'W' pattern may be seen else dominant 'S'.

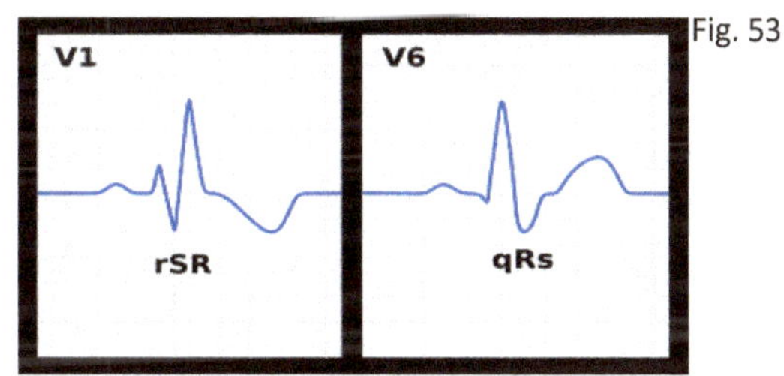

Fig. 53

In both RBBB & LBBB 'QRS' duration delayed (> 0.12 sec)

Conduction across the right bundle is blocked. So, right ventricular depolarization is delayed and does not start till the left ventricle is nearly entirely depolarized; so, ECG scribes, -

1. Delay of right ventricular depolarization extends the total time for ventricular depolarization. So, the QRS complex widens (> 0.12 seconds.

2. Wide QRS complex supposes an exclusive, almost diagnostic shape in leads superimposing right ventricle (V_1 V_2), where the normal QRS complex consists of a small R wave and a deep S wave, suggesting the electrical domination of left ventricle.

   In RBBB; initial R and S waves scribed, as left ventricle depolarizes but right ventricle initiates its delayed depolarization, unopposed by the now totally depolarized thus electrically quiet left ventricle. So, the electrical axis of current swings suddenly back to right and scribes second R wave called R' (R prime) in leads V_1 and V_2 forming RSR' complex looks like rabbit ears. On the other hand, in left lateral leads superimposing left ventricle (I, aVL, V_5, and V_6), late right ventricular depolarization scribes reciprocal late deep S waves.

➤ Incomplete Bundle Branch Block: ECG scribes RABBIT ears in V_1 as in RBBB but QRS between 0.10 to 0.12 seconds.

NORMAL	LBBB
Depolarization goes to left then right fascicles as refractory period of right fascicle is more → Ventricular septal activation responsible for the generation of 'q.' V_5 V_6 being the lateral leads and as the current goes away from V_5 V_6 towards V_1 V_2; 'q' which indicates septal activation shown in V_5 V_6 normally.	As Left fascicle is damaged → depolarization current takes more time to propagate (as refractory period of left is now > right) → 'q' will not develop in V_5 V_6, rather taller 'R' developed. • **Absent of 'q' in V_5 V_6** • Tall 'R' in V_5 V_6 with 'RABBIT EAR' appearance (due to inter-myocytic conduction with sequential activation of ventricle instead of simultaneous activation). • Deep 'S' in V_1 V_2

The main pathophysiological concern is sequential activation of ventricles instead of simultaneous activation → ventricles contract independently of each other → pulling of blood in lungs → PULMONARY HYPERTENSION.

As the Depolarization is abnormal so also the Repolarization → NON-DISCORDANT 'ST' elevation & 'T' wave changes.

It implies the fact that, the 'ST' segment change is always* occur "**Opposite of that of the DOMINANT 'QRS' vector**" → So, ST/T move opposite of the predominant 'QRS' → Deep 'S' in precordial (V_1V_2) leads with 'ST' elevation & in lateral (V_5V_6) leads - tall 'R' with 'ST' depression. QRS duration also increase (> 0.12 sec.) as in Ventricular tachycardia.

So, in a nutshell, **"Broad QRS in V_1V_2, Normal HR, absent of 'q' in V_5V_6, 'ST' elevation, Failure of 'R' progression, tall T', 'W-pattern' in V_1 & 'M-pattern' in V_6 (WilliaM) confirms LBBB**.

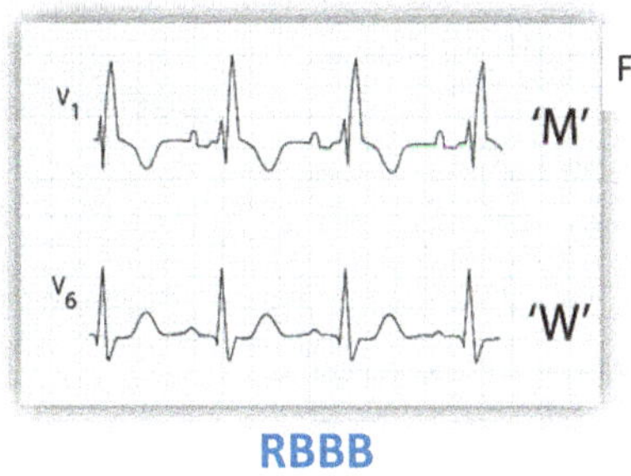

Fig. 54a

RBBB

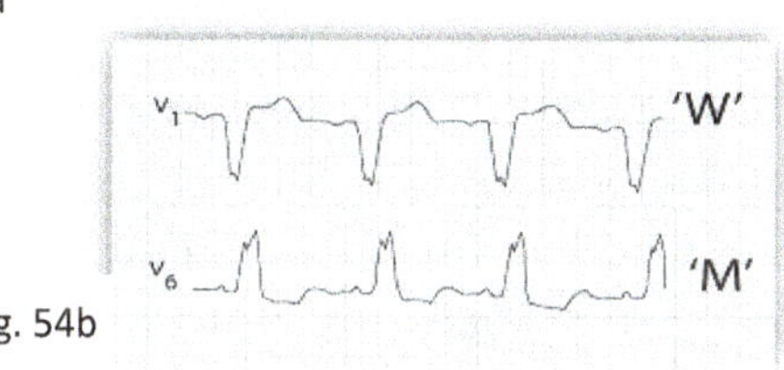

Fig. 54b

LBBB

- RSR' pattern in $V_1 V_2$
- Dominant 'S' in $V_5 V_6$

As ventricle contracts here → no chance of Pulmonary HTN; so harmless if not complicated by other issues.

- Dominant (deep) 'S' in $V_1 V_2$
- Tall 'R' in $V_5 V_6$
- Absent of 'q' in $V_5 V_6$ (usually)
- If found 'rabbit ear' pattern – significant but not always present
- Can occur in MI and may mimic MI → leads to Pulmonary HTN

➤ Non-specific INTRAventricular conduction delay: When there is QRS widening > 0.1 seconds without any criteria of Bundle Branch Block or Bifascicular block.

CAUSES

RBBB	LBBB

RBBB

Physiological
RVH
Pulmonary embolism
Cor pulmonale
IHD
RHD
Cardiomyopathy (e.g., in DM-II)

LBBB

A2: Aortic Stenosis, Ant. wall MI
D2: Digoxin toxicity, dilated cardiomyopathy (also cause of Ventricular bigeminy)
H2: HTN, Hyperkalemia

Critical Rate in Bundle Branch Block

Both RBBBs and LBBBs can be intermittent or permanent. In some cases, BBB appears only when a certain higher heart rate (tachycardia), the **critical rate** is achieved. So, ventricles perform normally at normal heart rates but above a certain rate, BBB develops. The development of a rate-related BBB is directly related to the time it requires a particular bundle branch to repolarize and thus make itself prepared for the next impulse to arrive. However, as the rate slows down, normalcy returns a bit lower than the critical rate.

If the heart rate is so fast, that a particular bundle branch cannot repolarize in time, there will be a temporary block to conduction, resulting in the classic ECG appearance of a rate-related BBB.

Incidence of rate-related BBB regulated by the same physiology, which reasons for aberrant conduction of supraventricular arrhythmias, in which the aberrantly conducted supraventricular beat results from some portion of the bundle branch system fail to repolarize in time.

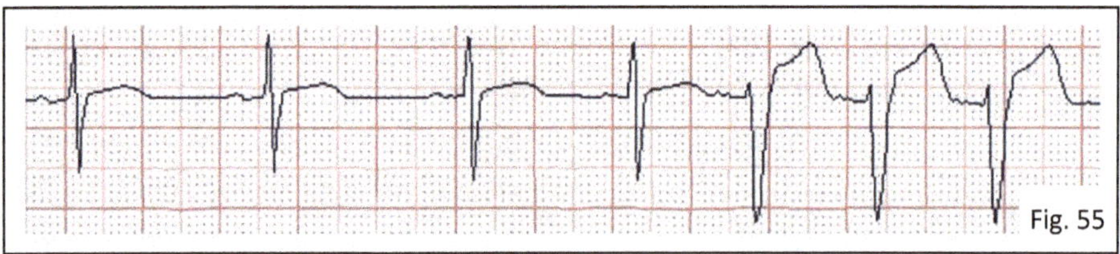

Fig. 55

Paradoxical Critical Rate (Bradycardia dependent BBB)

In case of real or relative bradycardia, BBB develops; as sinus rhythms are repeatedly interrupted by atrial extrasystoles. All the conducted beats to ventricles ending the stretched cycles following extrasystole beats show RBBB.

♥ HEMIBLOCK

– obviously exclusive to Left Bundle Branch as only Left BB have branches (fascicles).

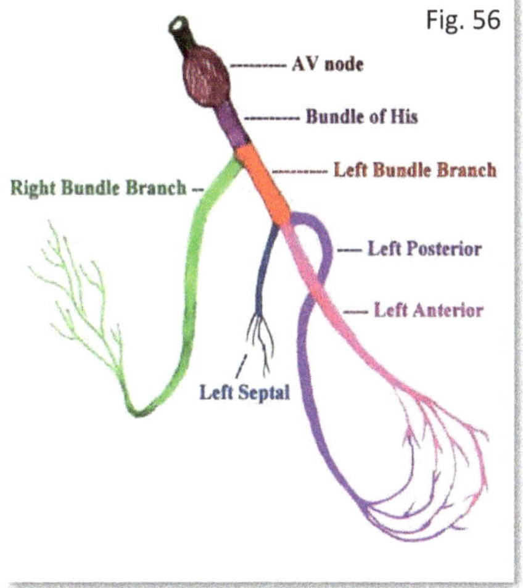

Left Bundle Branch divided in three fascicles Anterior, Posterior & Septal.

The major effect that hemiblocks imprint on ECG is AXIS DEVIATION.

The left anterior fascicle lies superiorly and laterally to the left posterior fascicle.

LEFT ANTERIOR HEMIBLOCK

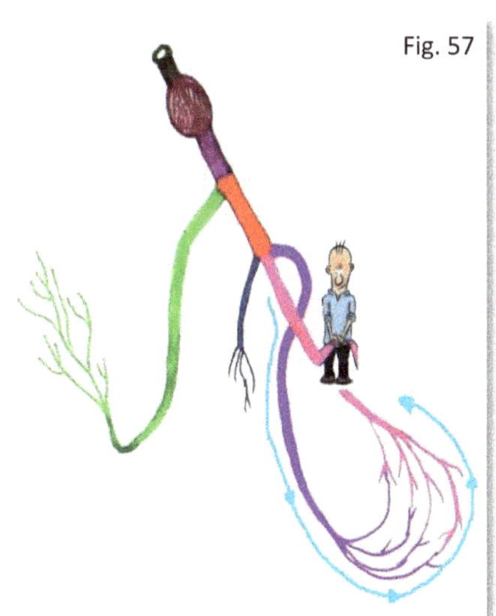

Here, the conduction down the left anterior fascicle is blocked.

All the current for that reason flows down the left posterior fascicle to the inferior surface of the heart. Left ventricular myocardial depolarization then occurs, progressing in an inferior-to-superior and right-to-left direction. The axis of ventricular depolarization is therefore redirected upward and slightly leftward, imprinting **tall positive R** waves **in the left lateral leads** and **deep S** waves **inferiorly**.

This results in **left axis deviation** in which the electrical axis of ventricular depolarization is redirected between −30° and −90°.

The easiest method is to look at the QRS complex in leads I and aVF. The QRS complex will be positive in lead I and negative in lead aVF − this analysis ensures axis range from 0° to −90°. Now lead II, which is angled at +60°; if QRS complex is negative, then axis more negative than −30°.

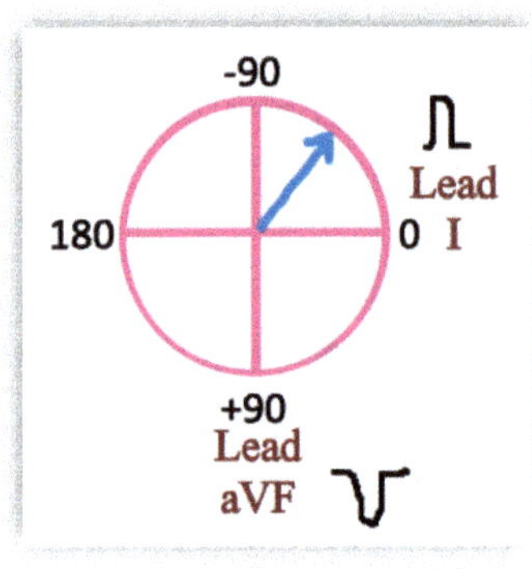

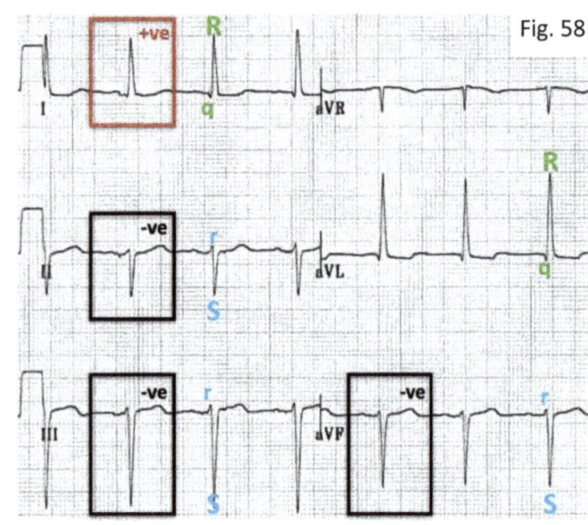

Fig. 58

LEFT POSTERIOR HEMIBLOCK

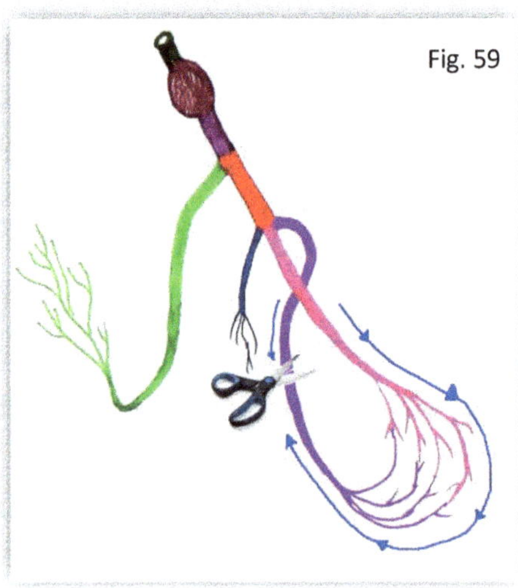
Fig. 59

In left posterior hemiblock, reversal occurs. All the current rushes down the left anterior fascicle and ventricular myocardial depolarization ensues in a superior-to-inferior and left-to-right direction.

So, the axis of depolarization is directed downward and rightward, imprinting **tall R waves inferiorly and deep S waves in the left lateral leads**.

The result is **right axis deviation** (i.e., the electrical axis of ventricular depolarization is between +90° and 180°). The QRS complex will be negative in lead I and positive in lead aVF.

Fig. 60

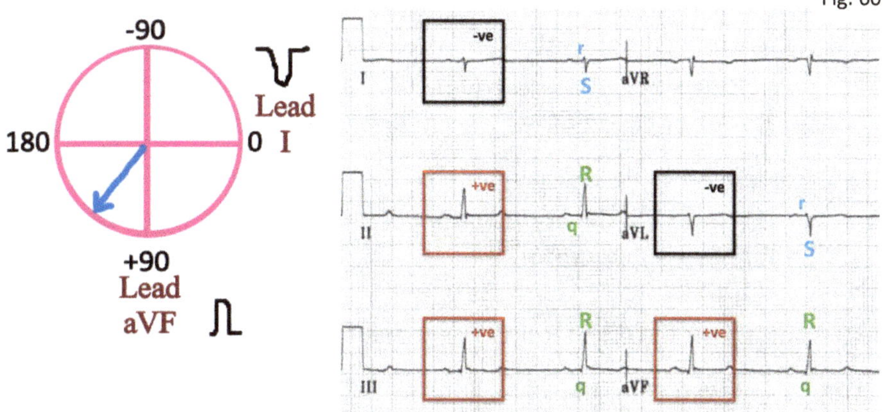

GENERAL CONSIDERATION OF HEMIBLOCK

Note: Hemiblocks <u>do not prolong</u> the QRS complex, which is widened in complete left and right bundle branch block. QRS duration in both left anterior and left posterior hemiblocks is near <u>normal</u>. There are no ST-segment and T wave changes also. **Left anterior hemiblock (LAHB)** is far **more common** than left posterior hemiblock, having extended but lighter and has a feebler blood supply than the posterior fascicle assumed to be the cause.

LAHB can be seen in both normal and diseased hearts! Whereas left posterior hemiblock is almost the sole domain of a sick heart.

D/D: Before confirming hemiblock, it is always necessary to make sure about the absence of other causes of axis deviation (e.g., ventricular hypertrophy). Patients with certain clinical disorders (e.g., severe COPD) can develop right axis deviation. However, for most patients, if the ECG is normal except for the presence of axis deviation, it is almost sure that hemiblock is present.

➤ **HEMIBLOCK in a nutshell**

Hemiblock is diagnosed by looking for left or right axis deviation.

Left Anterior Hemiblock:
1. Normal QRS duration and no ST-segment or T wave changes.
2. Left axis deviation between −30° and −90°.
3. No other cause of left axis deviation is present.

Left Posterior Hemiblock:
1. Normal QRS duration and no ST-segment or T wave changes.
2. Right axis deviation.

BIFASCICULAR BLOCKS: RBBB + any one fork of LBB (Hemiblock)

RBBB + Left Anterior HemiBlock:
- ✓ RBBB: QRS > 0.12 sec. + RSR' in V_1 and V_2
- ✓ LAHB: LAD between −30∘ and −90∘

RBBB + Left Posterior HemiBlock:
- ✓ RBBB: QRS > 0.12 sec. + RSR' in V_1 and V_2
- ✓ LPHB: RAD

♥ **PACEMAKER and ECG**

Current from pacemaker scribes on ECG as small 'spike'.

1. Atrial pacemaker : Generates 'spike' followed by 'P' with normal PR interval and normal QRS pattern being supraventricular.

   These patients often show 1∘ AV block or Wenckebach conduction on their paced ECG, which is not apparent on their baseline tracing as they commonly have some degree of AV node dysfunction (e.g., due to age-related AV-nodal degeneration / underlying cardiac issue / post-operative ischemia / AV-nodal blocking medications).

   When paced at a faster rate than AV node can manage → "exhausted" → 1∘ AV block or Wenckebach phenomenon on the paced ECG.

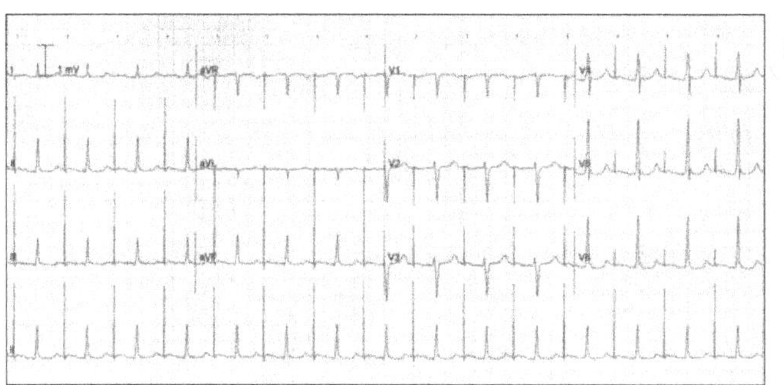

Atrial paced rhythm with 1° AV block

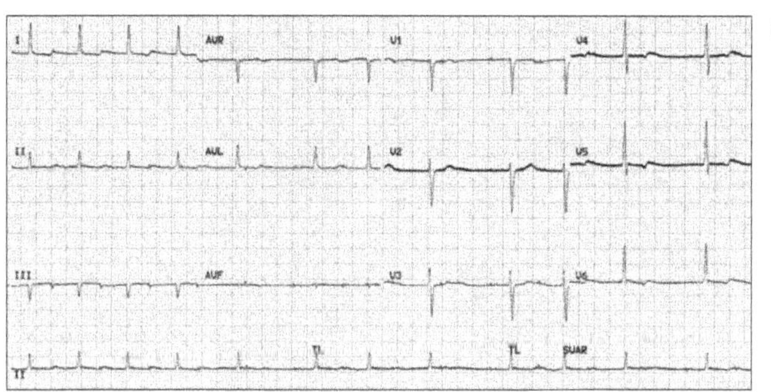

Atrial paced rhythm with Wencheback (MT-I)

2. Ventricular pacemaker : QRS is wide and bizarre (not normal path – as electrode placed in right ventricle, which depolarizes earlier than left as in LBBB; a retrograde 'P' may be found.

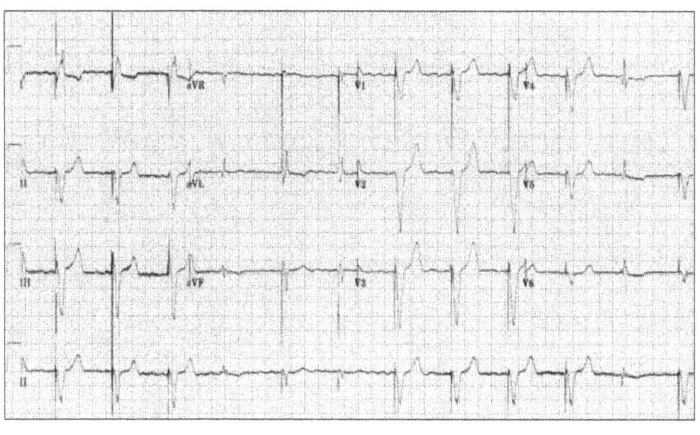

3. Dual Chamber, AV sequential pacemaker : QRS is wide and bizarre (not normal path, as elctrode placed in right ventricle, which depolarizes earlier than left as in LBBB; a retrograde 'P' may scribe.

Both atrial and ventricular pacing spikes are visible before each QRS complex. Small P waves are seen following each atrial pacing spike and a QRS complex follows each ventricular pacing spike. QRS complexes are broad with a LBBB pattern, indicating the presence of a ventricular pacing electrode in the right ventricle.

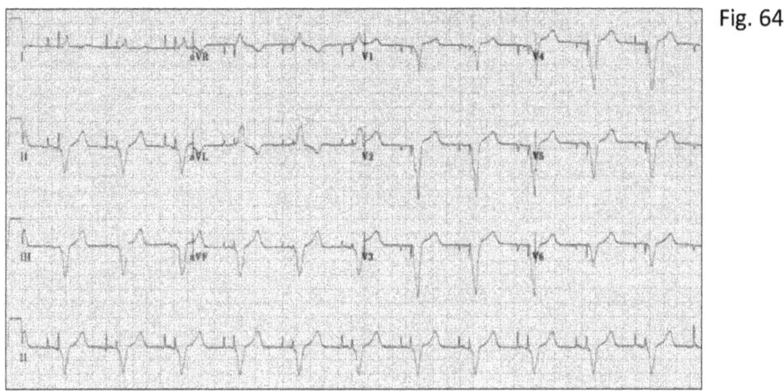

Fig. 64

ECG with wide QRS and LAD must always be suspected the presence of pacemaker, as pacemaker spikes cannot be seen if less than 1 mV.

<u>NOTE</u>

🫀 ⑤ Precocious marvel!

Board honors 5-year-old student for her reading milestones

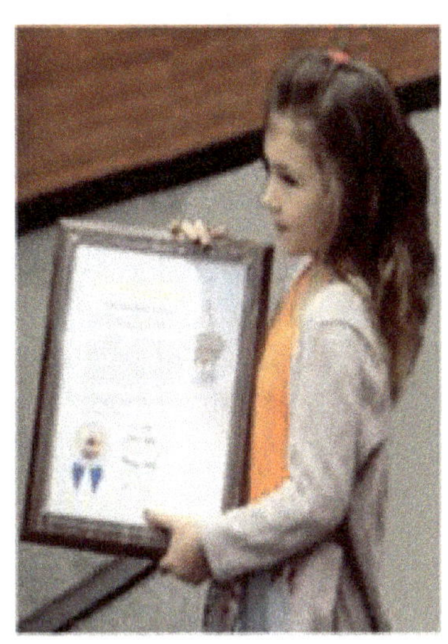

..... precocious Missouri native loves to read books each and every day. Sternemann's passion led her to become a participant in the 1,000 Books Before Kindergarten Campaign, a nonprofit group that partners with participating local libraries to encourage literacy in young children, ranging from infants to toddlers. She performed a significant achievement by completing the campaign three times, reading 1,000 books in her hometown of St. Louis and 2,000 books in Apollo Beach, where she and her parents reside. ......

News posted 20th January 2023

Photo information: The Hillsborough County Board of County Commissioners present a commendation to five-year-old Liandromeda Stememann.

Preexcitation / precociousness in study being a bibliophile is impressive, but Preexcitation in cardiac electrical event may even lead to death.

❤ PREEXCITATION SYNDROMEs

Here, conducting current reach ventricles from atria earlier than usual. In normal conduction, major delay is at the AV node, where the depolarization current held nearly for 0.1 second to facilitate atria to pour most blood to ventricles. Otherwise, in preexcitation syndromes there are accessory abnormally conducting pathways, through which the current bypass AV node and arrives ventricles in earlier time.

1. Louis **Wolff**-John **Parkinson**-Paul Dudley **White syndrome**:

An unusual faster pathway between atria and ventricles bypassing AV node (e.g., bundle of Kent) → depolarization wave bypass the AV delay and reach ventricles faster → ECG scribes PR interval < 0.12 seconds; … and eventually fused with the wave coming through normal (AV nodal) pathway → slurred upsloping at beginning of the QRS complex scibed in ECG called 'delta wave'.

Fig. 65

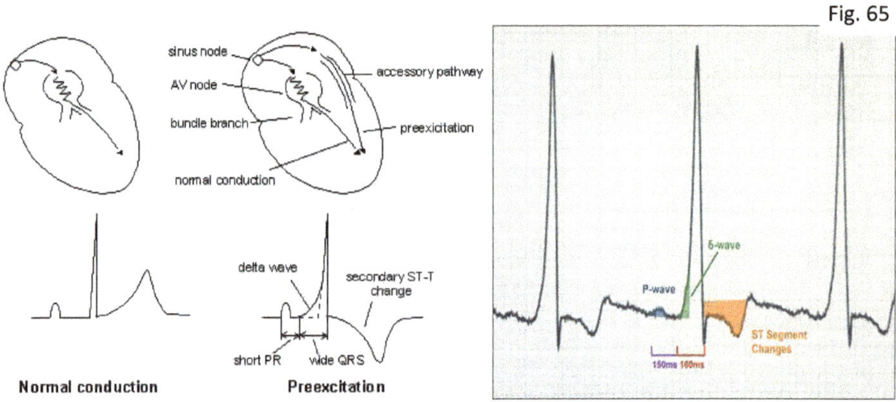

This may initiate tachycardia with exiting factors (coffee, anxiety, alcohol, exercise, etc.) → focus near bundle of Kent → Re-entry ensues → dangerous tachycardia (is also called AV Reciprocating Tachycardia, **AVRT**).

Tachycardia activate ventricles in an antegrade maner through AV node → narrow QRS complex.

Atrial fibrillation in WPW: It is ominous, the accessory path acts as free conduit for the chaotic atrial activity, practically it is like without AV node state and ventricular rate rise as high as 300 bpm:

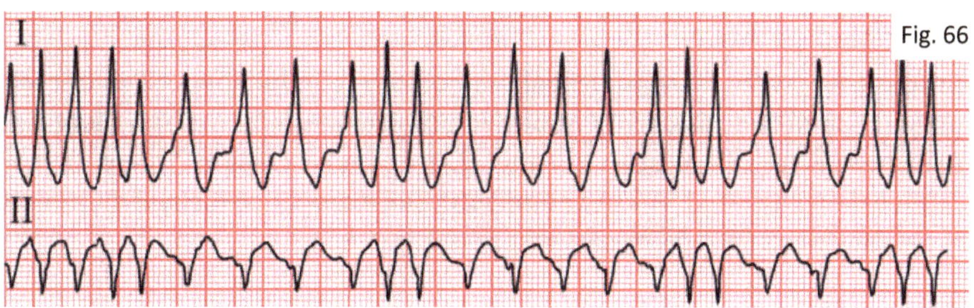

Very irregular tachycardia, no visible P, most QRS are wide having slurred upstroke

So, briefly we get:

- PR interval < 120ms.
- Delta wave: slurring slow rise of initial portion of the QRS.
- QRS prolongation > 110ms.
- Discordant ST-segment and T wave changes (i.e., in the opposite direction to the major component of the QRS complex).
- Pseudo-infarction pattern in up to 70% of patients — due to negatively deflected delta waves in inferior/anterior leads ("pseudo-Q waves"), or prominent R waves in V1-3 (mimicking posterior infarction).

An AP can conduct impulses in three ways:
- **In both directions** (common).
- **Retrograde only**, away from the ventricle (15%).
- **Anterograde only**, towards the ventricle (rare).

The direction of conduction affects the appearance of the ECG in sinus rhythm and during tachyarrhythmias. APs can be **left-sided** or **right-sided**, and ECG features will vary depending on this:
- Left-sided AP: produces a positive delta wave in all precordial leads, with $R/S > 1$ in V_1. Sometimes referred to as a **type A WPW pattern**.
- Right-sided AP: produces a negative delta wave in leads V_1 and V_2. Sometimes referred to as a **type B WPW pattern**.

Note that the features of pre-excitation may be subtle, or present only intermittently. Pre-excitation may be more pronounced with increased vagal tone e.g., during Valsalva maneuvers, or with AV blockade e.g., drug therapy.

Concealed pathway

In patients with retrograde-only accessory conduction, all anterograde conduction occurs via the AV node. No pre-excitation occurs and therefore no features of WPW are seen on the ECG in sinus rhythm. This is termed a "concealed pathway." These patients can still experience tachyarrhythmias, as the pathway can still form part of a re-entry circuit.

2. Lown-**G**anong-**L**evine **syndrome**:

Congenitally presence of accessory pathway which connects atria to ventricles bypassing AV node. In WPW accessory path connects to ventricular myocardium but in LGL it connects with normal pathway (Bundle of His). In LGL no delta wave and may initiate PSVT.

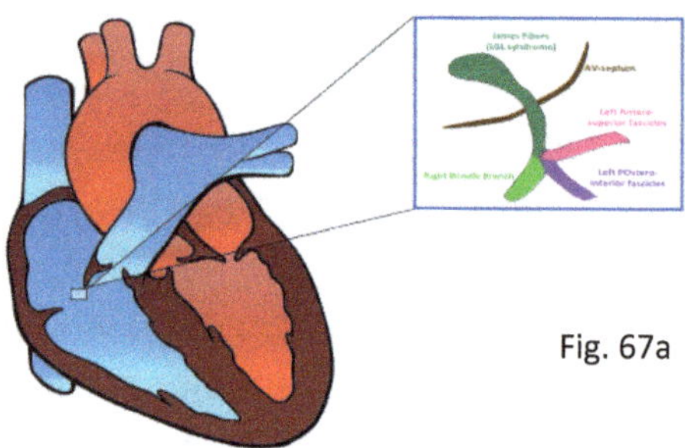

Fig. 67a

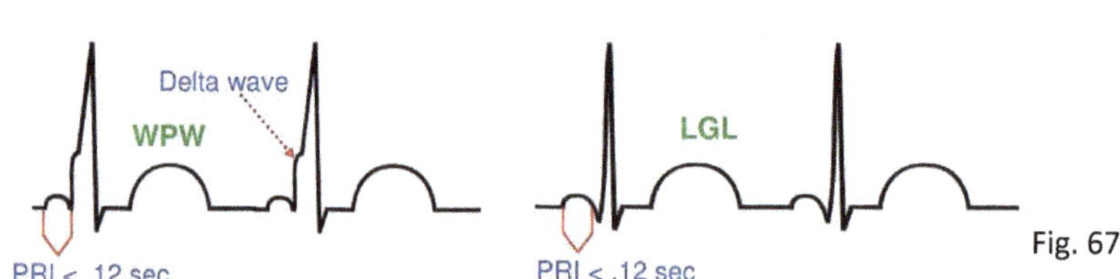

Fig. 67b

Now, if by any means AV start conducting fast (e.g. sympathomimetic as intake of caffeine, alcohol, anxiety, etc.) → **Ectopic foci** fires → current pass through Bundle of Kent → current go downwards as well as re-enters through AV-JT (while no current coming down through AV) and reach previous situ while in re-excitable state (every 0.4 sec.) → Rotating (like re-entry) → JUNCTIONAL TACHYCARDIA [similarly also due to INTRANODAL PHENOMENON (when in AV node one slow and another fast conducting pathway present)].

💔 With accessory pathways, the axis and or amplitude usually change; so, in presense of those determining BBB or Hypertrophy may be questionable.

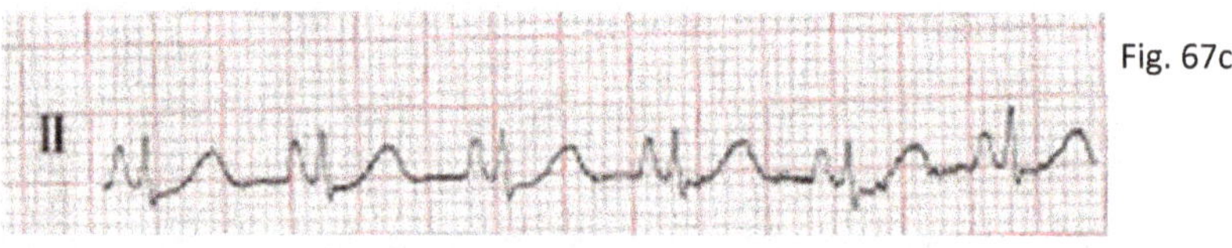

Fig. 67c

LGL syndrome with P-R interval = or < 0.08 second in lead II

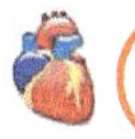 # ⑥ Stagnation is death

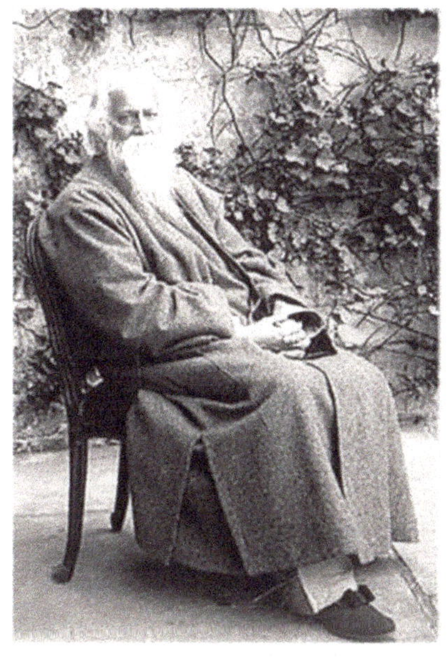

দুই উপমা

যে নদী হারায়ে স্রোত চলিতে না পারে

সহস্র শৈবালদাম বাঁধে আসি তারে;

যে জাতি জীবনহারা অচল অসাড়

পদে পদে বাঁধে তারে জীর্ণ লোকাচার।

সর্বজন সর্বক্ষণ চলে যেই পথে

তৃণগুল্ম সেথা নাহি জন্মে কোনোমতে;

যে জাতি চলে না কভু তারি পথ-'পরে

তন্ত্র-মন্ত্র-সংহিতায় চরণ না সরে।

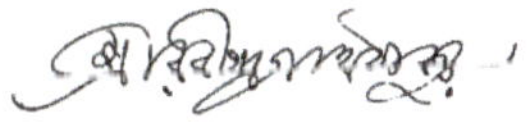

The river that cannot flow without a stream,
enclosed by a thousand algae-cream.

The nation that has lost its life is anchored, bind
step by step with worn-out mood.

Everyone always on the way,
grass is not born in any way.

The nation, not follow its direction ever,
cannot move on by magical interfere.

* Thought translation

Noble laureate "World-poet" – Rabindranath Tagore

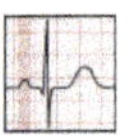 # Myocardial Ischemia and infarction

[Iskhaimos (Gk.) "stanching or stopping blood," from iskhein "to hold, curb, keep back, restrain" + haima "blood"]

Ischemia refers to a lack of oxygen due to inadequate perfusion.

Ischemic heart disease is a condition resulted by various causes, all having in common a disruption of cardiac function due to an **IMBALANCE BETWEEN OXYGEN SUPPLY AND DEMAND**.

This lack of oxygen supply to myocardium scribes 'T wave' changes.

ANGINA ("I cry" = weeping of myocardium due to want of food!)

It is chest pain, due to the relative deficit of oxygen between demand and supply. The classical symptom of myocardial ischemia represented as diffused chest pain with opression, heaviness and often associated with dizziness, SOB, nausea, vomiting to sweating. It may remain stable for years or if an ominous situation, may precipitate infarction. During acute attack ECG scribes ST-segment depression or T wave inversion.

Some patients' myocardium only cry during work, climbing stairs, even in little work; but not while in rest, which is called 'Angina on Effort.' For this reason, a resting ECG reveals no abnormality. To elicit this the patient must undergo 'Stress test;' ECG while running on a treadmill setup to unveil hidden evil part (provoked angina).

Not every angina only bought or aggravated by effort! Some anginas can even occur anytime, even at rest – prinzmetal angina. This occurs due to vasospasm of coronary artery. ECG scribes ST-segment elevation.

Ischemia is usually reversible and on return of balance between supply and demand, leaves no residual damage. T wave changes come to normal; whereas infarction leads to tissue destruction due to prolonged disruption of blood supply to myocardium; scribes T wave inversion even for years.

T wave inversion is very <u>non-specific</u> finding for infarction but usually indicates ischemia; though various other issues like BBB, Ventricular hypertrophy ('strain') with repolarization abnormality, HOCM, Pulmonary embolism, CNS infarct/Sub-arachnoid bleeding, etc. can invert T wave. In ischemia, T inversion is symmetrical whereas in other issues there is slow usual descent but sharp ascent.

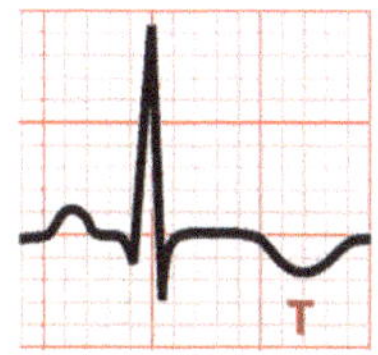

Fig. 68

'T wave' due to ischemia   'T wave' due to other causes

Patients having ECG already with T wave inversion as normally found in children /BBB /Ventricular strain /HOCM or raised intracranial pressure; ischemia may *'revert'* them to normal, called **pseudo-normalization**.

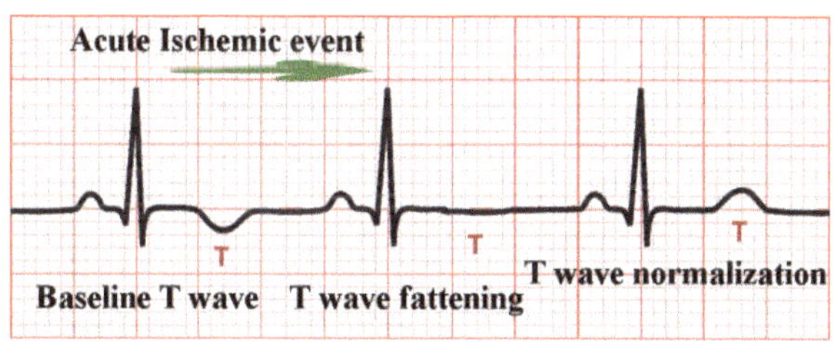

Fig. 69

> ➤ **ECG progresses in three stages in AMI (ST-Elevation MI)**

Stage-I   : T wave peaking

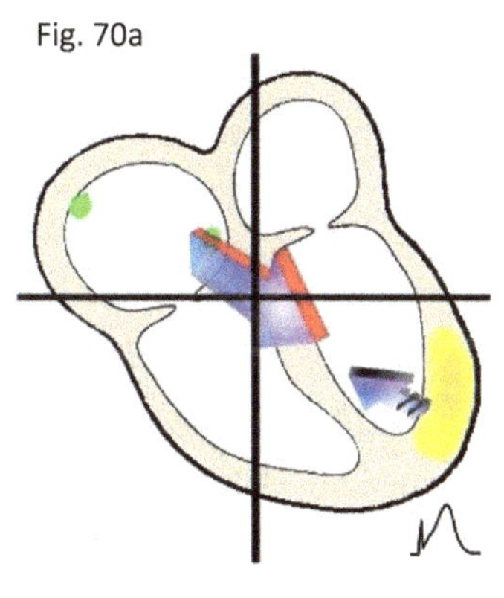

Fig. 70a

1. As repolarization is an *active* process, which need energy and 'repolarization' may be calculated as *'negative* depolarization'; so, T wave peaking may be due to strong quicker repolarizaton as the function of the pumps increased and cation influx /

2. Depolarization that is going on, is comparatively stronger → adding two unidirectional vectors (negative coming + positive going).

Stage-II : T wave inversion

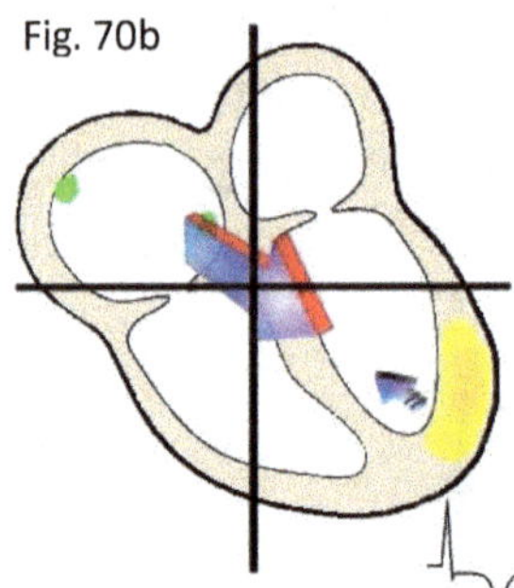

Fig. 70b

Ischemia → inflammation increased → passive pouring diminished + voltage gated pumps non/less-functioning → K$^+$ efflux started but less influx → hyperacute polarization → more negativity.

Stage-III : ST-segment elevation and formation of deep Q wave

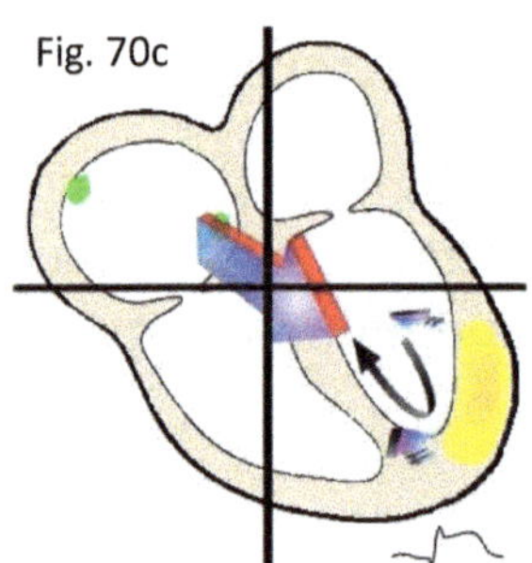

Fig. 70c

Current can't pass through dead myocytes (act as a-electric / insulator) → so healthy portions depolarizes first (going away from lead II) → ST elevation occur.

Died myocardium became electronically silent → current directed away → deep negative deflection Q wave scribed.

Fig. 71

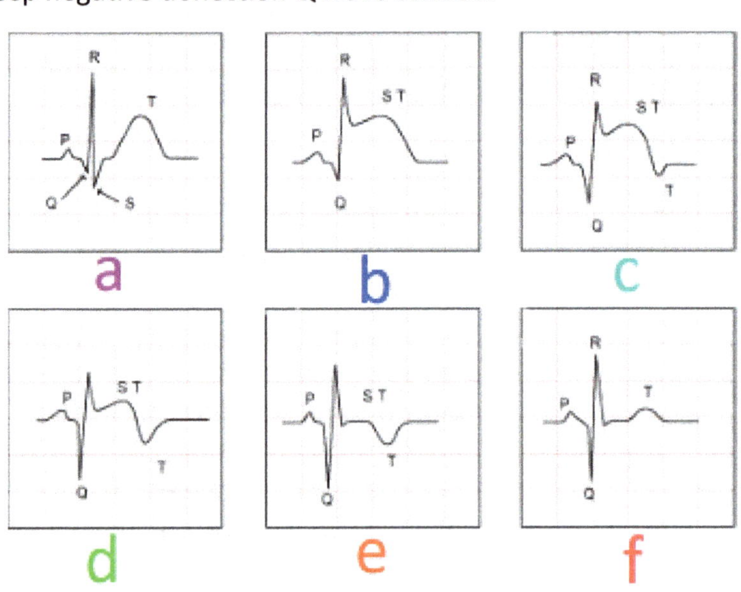

Fig. 71(a) – It shows a normal sinus complex. The ST-segment is on the iso-electric line. At the onset of pain, the ECG is normal, but the ST-segment soon begin to alter. Here, the T wave is peaked.

Fig. 71(b) – Within an hour, ST-segment markedly elevated; denoting, onset of myocardial necrosis. In this situation, thrombolytic drug administered.

Fig. 71(c) – On administration of thrombolytic, there are definite changes as 50% drop in ST-segment elevation than Fig. 70(b) is seen, which bears good prognosis. These changes usually occur within ninety minutes of administering thrombolytics. There may be much deeper 'U wave inversion,' a good sign of reperfusion.

Fig. 71(d) – A Day later, the ST-segment mostly returns to iso-electric line, but the T wave remains inverted. It may stay inverted for days to even months.

Fig. 71(e & f) – In some cases, after a few months the ECG looks relatively normal. Compare picture 6 with Fig. 70(a). They look much the same but the deep Q wave in Fig. 70(f). **A deep Q wave is an indicator of myocardial tissue death (old infarct) and will remain on the ECG.**

A "pathological" Q wave is not "time-specific". It may be there from a previous MI and therefore is not the criteria for evaluating an AMI.

T wave peaking is better indicator than serum potassium level! which can be mistaken with peaked T waves in AMI; in hyperkalemia, peaking seen universally (diffuse) almost all over instead of localization in AMI.

ST-segment elevation (STE) is also somewhat non-specific and found in other issues as in pericarditis, which cause ST-segment elevation with T wave flattening and inversion but usually diffusely unlike localized as in AMI, in pericarditis Q wave absent – we need a clinical evaluation too. In normal heart, if ST-segment elevation seen, referred as **J-point elevation** or *early repolarization*. Fig. 72 shows various J-points.

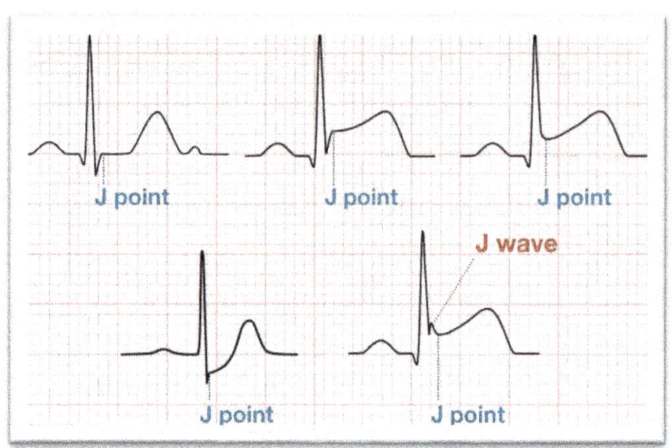

Fig. 72

J-point elevation is frequently found in healthy young individuals and ST-segment usually returns to baseline with exercise. ST-segment arched upward and tend to blend subtly with T wave in AMI, whereas in J-point elevation, T wave keeps distinct individuality.

As stated earlier, ST-segment usually returns to baseline within few hours of the event, whereas persistent ST-segment elevation may indicate **ventricular aneurysm**.

Reciprocal changes occur to the leads placed at some distance from the site of infarction, scribe tall positive R waves as well as ST-segment and T wave changes, leads to even as ST-segment depression; as current apparently twist toward those leads.

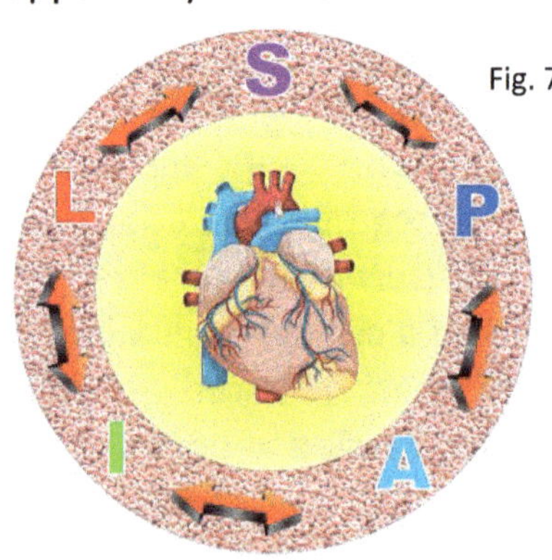

Fig. 73

This cycle "Septal ⟷ Posterior ⟷ Anterior ⟷ Inferior ⟷ Lateral ⟷ Septal" shown clock-wise, helps to find the reciprocal changes depending on the position of ST-segment elevation. The reciprocal changes are expected two adjascent zones.

Every Q wave is not abnormal. Small Q waves can be seen with absolute normal heart, in the left lateral leads and sometimes in the inferior leads, which signify the early left to right depolarization of interventricular septum. Infarction scribes wider and deeper Q waves, where *Q wave duration > 0.04 second and depth should ≥ 1/3 of the adjacent R wave*; except lead aVR, where normally deep Q waves present due to opposite position with major vector, so this lead spared to consider for infarction.

Now, with all the above armaments, localization of the infarct is crucial to enumerate therapeutic approches and prognostic implications.

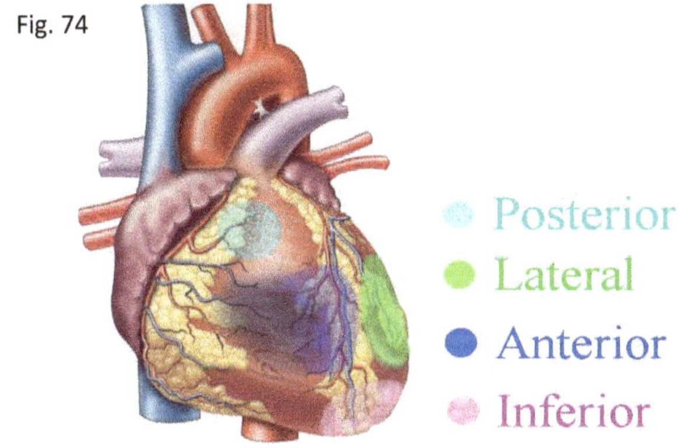

Fig. 74

> ## NON-Q wave MI

Not all MI produce Q waves. It was previously thought that the production of Q wave required full thickness (transmural) infarction of myocardial wall; and an absence of Q waves indicated a partial infarction, only to the inner layer (subendocardial). Though this is not perfect. So, better, to describe as 'Q wave-infarction' and 'non-Q wave-infarction.' So, the only ECG finding in cases of 'non-Q wave-infarction' is T wave inversion and ST-segment depression. Yes! 'ST-depression.'

Both angina and non-Q wave MI scribe ST-segment depression. But in angina the ST-segment touches baseline as soon as attack subside, whereas in MI, ST-segment remain depressed at least two days. Clinical features are different and cardiac markers are elevated in the MI cases.

Special Consideration with LBBB

Diagnosis of MI is too difficult in the patients with preexisting LBBB. As there is already 'ST' with abnormal 'T' elevation and chance of mistake is always remain, where "Sgarbossa criteria" have solution with reasonable specificity > 98% but low sensitivity < 20%, Total points ≥ 3:

Original "SGARBOSSA criteria" for Diagnosis of STEMI in LBBB   Fig. 75a

CRITERIA	POINTS	Normal LBBB	Ischemic LBBB
1. CONCORDANCE ST-ELEVATION ≥ 1 mm in ≥ one lead	5	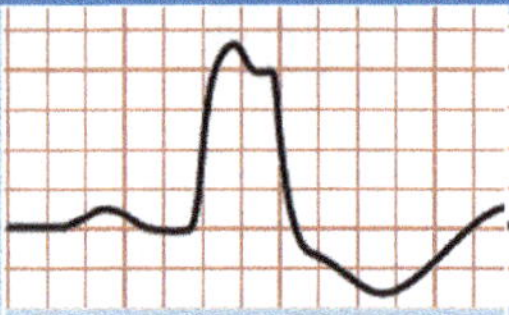	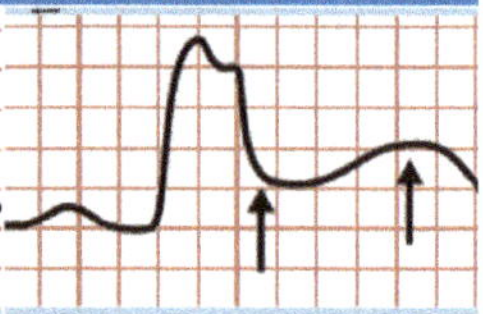
2. CONCORDANCE ST-DEPRESSION ≥ 1 mm in ≥ one lead of V$_1$, V$_2$, V$_3$	3	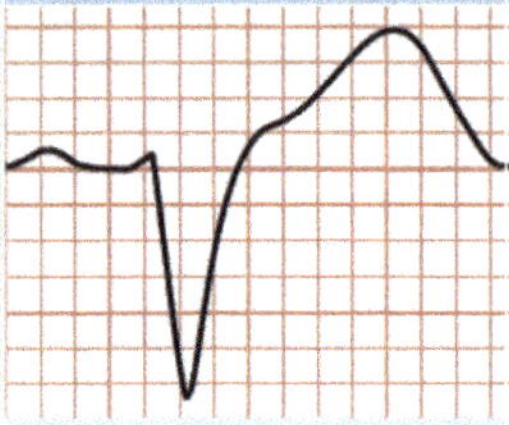	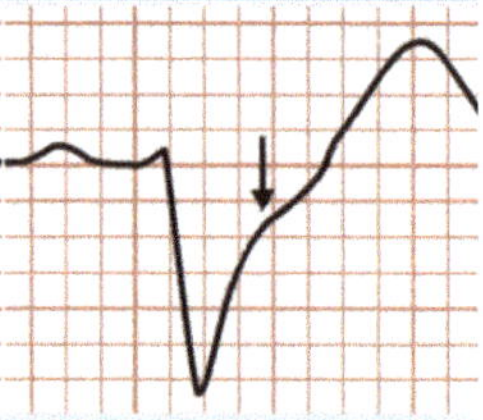
3. DISCORDANCE ST-ELEVATION > 5 mm in ≥ one lead	2	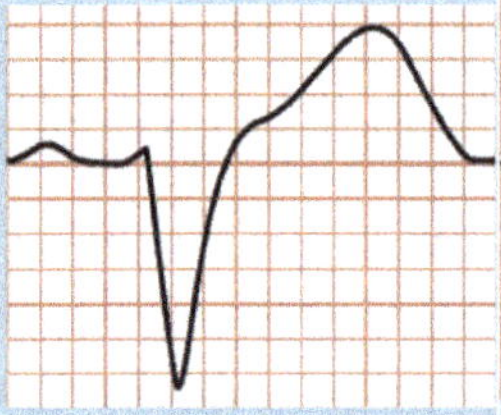	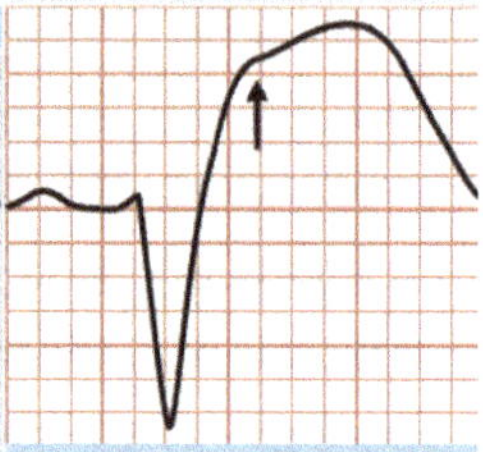

"SMITH" modified "SGARBOSSA criteria"

Dr. Smith modified "Sgarbossa criteria" increased its sensitivity many fold. Where there is a change only in the 3rd criterion as:

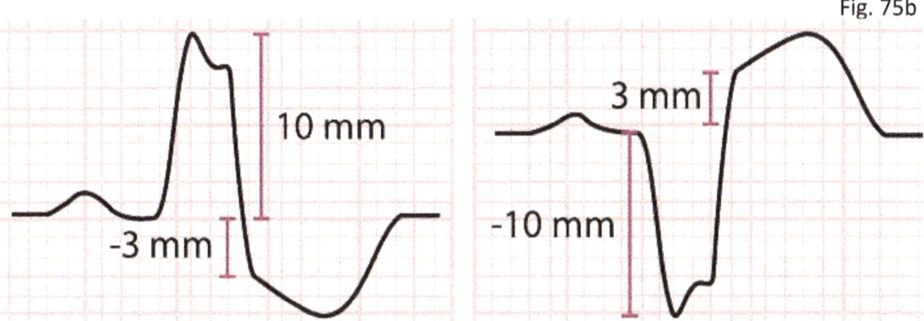

'Proportionally EXCESSIVE discordent STE in ≥ 1 lead anywhere with ≥ 1 mm STE, as defined by ≥ 25% (1/4th) of the depth of preceding S wave.

In nutshell, MI diagnoses based on the history of present illness; as sudden onset of long crushing, piercing retrosternal chest pain radiating to jaws, shoulders, left arm, concomitant with nausea, SOB, and diaphoresis.

CHEST LEAD PLACEMENTS OTHER THAN CONVENTIONAL

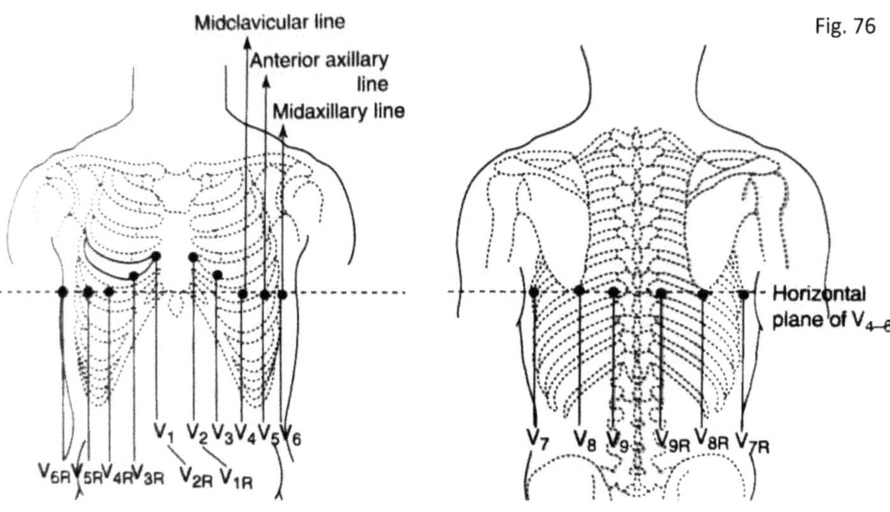

NOTE

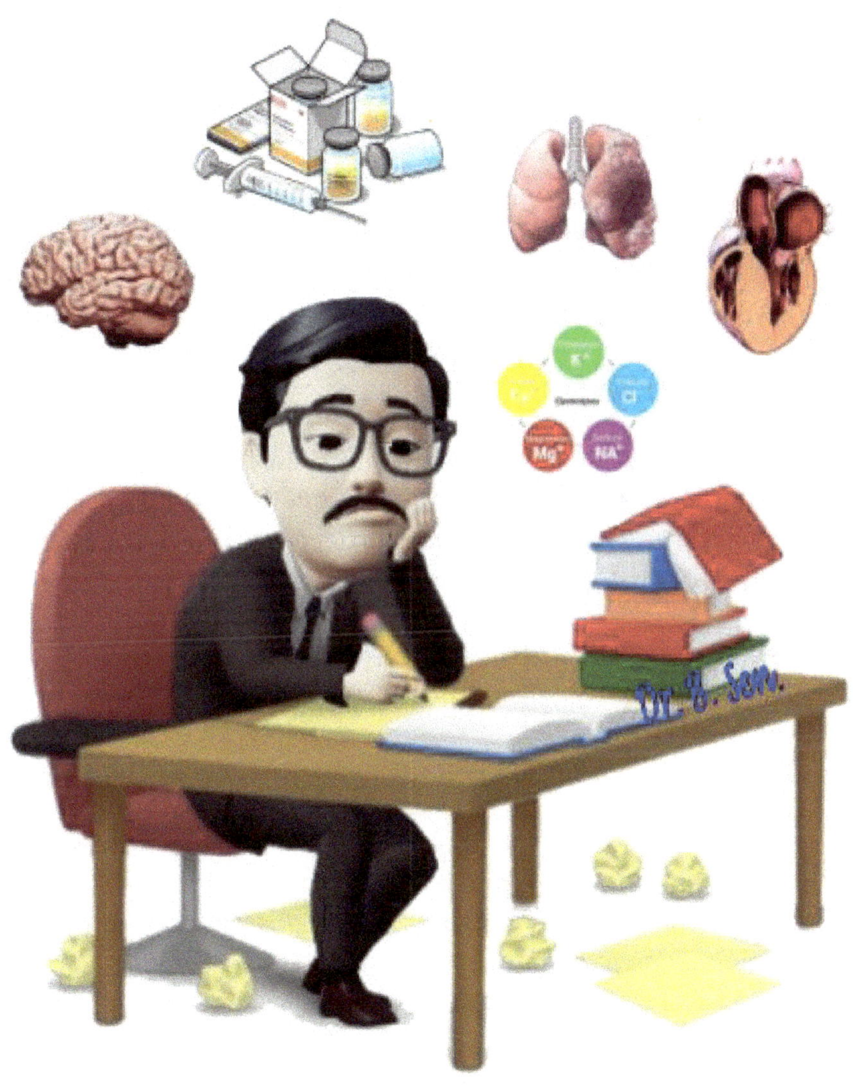

1. ANXIETY

   Tako-tsubo syndrome / Broken Heart Syndrome: In elderly women in emotional or physical stress, persuades reversible left ventricular dysfunction of a specific pattern extending beyond the region supplied by one coronary artery (usually, parts of the anterior wall and apical region) giving the appearance of a Japanese octopus pot, the Tako-tsubo; results in chest pain, hospitalization, even with cardiogenic shock. The admission ECG shows ST segment elevation in leads V_3–V_6, evolving in 3 days to deep T wave inversion, T wave flattening, and then further deepening at 2–3 weeks. Cardiac specific enzyme rise is low and LV dysfunction improves $\leq$ 2 weeks.

2. CENTRAL NERVOUS SYSTEM

   Cerebral Infarction / subarachnoid bleeding → autonomic nervous system fires → sinus bradycardia and diffuse symmetrical deepest and widest T wave inversion with prominent U wave (cf. asymmetric T wave in ventricular hypertrophy)

Raised Intracranial Pressure
- Widespread giant T wave inversions (Cerebral T waves)
- Prolonged QT
- Bradycardia (Cushing reflex – denotes impending brainstem herniation

Other possible ECG changes that may be seen:
- ST segment elevation / depression — *this may mimic myocardial ischemia or pericarditis*
- Increased U wave amplitude
- Other rhythm disturbances: sinus tachycardia, junctional rhythms, premature ventricular contractions, atrial fibrillation

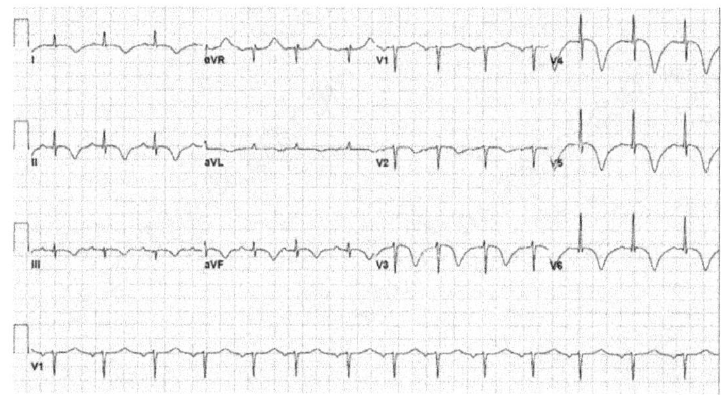

Fig. 77

Sinus rhythm with prolonged QT

3. ELECTROLYTE DISTURBANCES

Potassium

Hyperkalemia: Slightest change in ECG due to hyperkalemia dictates immediate intervention. Hyperkalemia produces a progressive evolution of changes that precipitate ominous ventricular fibrillation, which sometimes may be so tormenting, leads to sudden death.

ECG changes due to hyperkalemia have better clinical implication over serum potassium level! With the rise in potassium → ECG begin to peak proportionately and globally to all leads (c.f. in MI, it is confined to the leads overlying the area of infarction).

With further increase of serum potassium → PR interval becomes prolonged with gradual P wave flattening and later disappear → QRS-complex widens and then merges with the T wave → 'sinewave' pattern → Ventricular fibrillation developed.

Hypokalemia:

Hypokalemia is defined as a serum potassium level of < 3.5 mmol/L. ECG changes generally do not manifest until there is a moderate degree of hypokalemia (2.5-2.9 mmol/L). The earliest ECG manifestation of hypokalemia is a decrease in T wave amplitude.

ECG features of hypokalemia (K < 2.7 mmol/L)

- Increased P wave amplitude
- Prolonged PR-interval
- Widespread ST depression and T wave flattening / inversion
- Prominent U waves (V_2-V_3)
- Apparent long QT interval due to fusion of T and U waves (= long QU interval)

With worsening hypokalemia...

- Frequent supraventricular and ventricular ectopic
- Supraventricular tachyarrhythmias: AF, atrial flutter, atrial tachycardia
- Potential to develop life-threatening ventricular arrhythmias, e.g., VT, VF and Torsade de Pointes

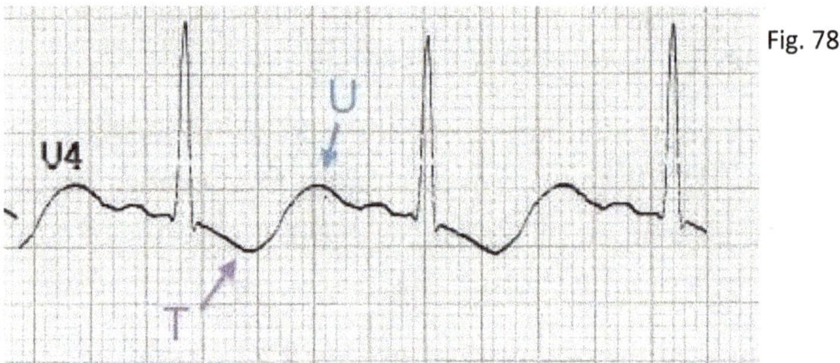

Hypokalemia: T wave inversion and prominent U waves

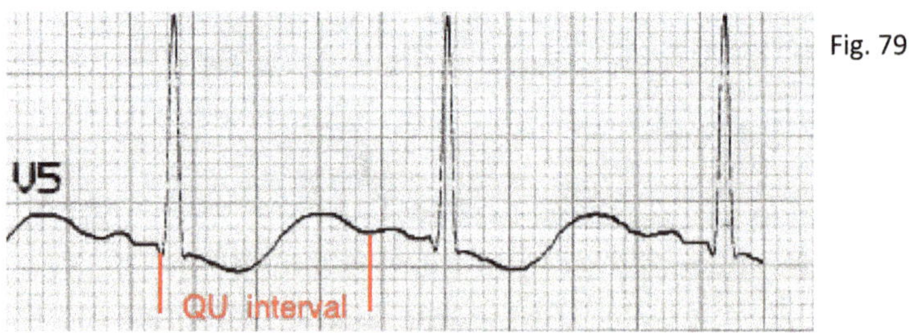

QU interval: The apparent pseudo-prolonged QT interval is the QU interval with an absent T wave.

The push-pull effect

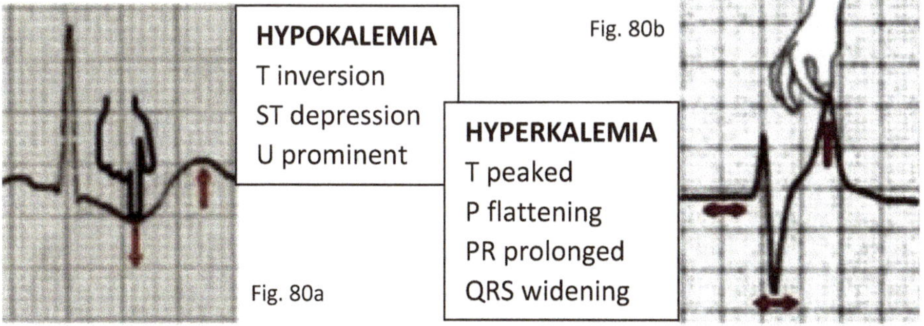

- Hypokalemia creates the illusion that the T wave is "pushed down," with resultant T wave flattening/inversion, ST depression, and prominent U waves
- In hyperkalemia, the T wave is "pulled upwards," creating tall "tented" T waves, and stretching the remainder of the ECG to cause P wave flattening, PR prolongation, and QRS widening

Pathophysiology

Potassium is vital for regulating the normal electrical activity of the heart. Decreased extracellular potassium causes myocardial hyperexcitability with the potential to develop re-entrant arrhythmias. ECG scribes ST-segment depression, flattening of T wave with prolongation of QT-interval and appearance of U wave. Though rarely, severe hypokalemia scribes ST-segment elevation too.

QT-interval if prolonged → a PVC falls on the prolonged T wave → torsade de pointes (also seen in hypocalcemia and hypomagnesemia).

Calcium

QT interval shortens in hypercalcemia and prolongs in hypocalcemia. Similar events like hypokalemia, i.e., torsade de pointes may precipitate. *As QT-interval normally varies with heart rate; corrected QT-interval used to assess the absolute QT-segment prolongation.*

4. HYPOTHERMIA

ECG reacts dynamically with a drop in body temperature. It seems to be a 'shutdown.'

a) Most confirmatory is ST-segment elevation, which is abrupt ascent right at the J-point and then equally sudden plunge back to baseline. This wave is known as 'J-wave' or 'Osborn wave.'
b) Sinus bradycardia along with prolongation of all segments and intervals.
c) Numerous arrhythmias may appear, in which s-l-o-w atrial fibrillation is commonest.
d) Muscle tremor artefact due to shivering in cold as also may found in Parkinson's disease, which should not be confused with atrial flutter.

5. THERAPEUTIC AGENTS

Digitalis

In therapeutic level: It produces **'digitalis effect'** as ST-segment depression with slow gradual downslope initializing subtly from the preceding R wave; along with T wave flattening, even inversion.

In toxic level: Sinus exit block or complete sinus node suppression may occur. In sick-sinus patients, even in therapeutic level it slows sinus rhythm. It also slows down conduction through AV node and causes all types of AV blocks. Enhanced automaticity of every conducting cell can initiate every type of tachyarrhythmia; PAT with 2nd° (2:1) AV block and PVC are the commonest among them.

Therapeutic agents that prolong QT-interval

Antiarrhythmic medicines (amiodarone, quinidine, etc.) are used to treat arrhythmia by prolonging QT-interval and paradoxically increase the risk of ominous ventricular fibrillation.

Commonly prescribed drugs have the capability to prolong QT-interval. Antibiotics (azithromycin, ciprofloxacin, erythromycin, levofloxacin, etc.); Antifungals (itraconazole, ketoconazole, etc.); Antihistamines (cetirizine, astemizole, etc.); Psychotropics (haloperidol, phenothiazine, etc.); Antidepressant (amitriptyline, etc.) and more.

Taking more than one agent at a time, need very close monitoring else it ultimately may precipitate torsade de pointes and death.

$$QTc = \frac{QT}{\sqrt{RR}}$$

[QTc should be < 500ms during treatment expect BBB where it must be < 550 ms]

 OTHER CARDIAC AND PERICARDIAL DISORDERS

Myocarditis: like other diffuse inflammatory processes, Conduction blocks, usually BBB and hemiblocks scribed in ECG.

HOCM: ECG is usually normal, few cases scribe features of LVH and LAD. Q waves may be found laterally and inferiorly (reciprocal changes). Apical HCM shows **giant T wave inversion** In the **precordial**, also in inferior and lateral leads. Localized hypertrophy of LV apex, causing an "ace of spades" configuration of the LV cavity on ventriculography.

PERICARDITIS:

- Widespread concave ST elevation and PR depression throughout most of the limb leads (I, II, III, aVL, aVF) and precordial leads (V2-6)
- Reciprocal ST depression and PR elevation in lead aVR (± V1)
- Sinus tachycardia is also common in acute pericarditis due to pain and/or pericardial effusion

NB: ST- and PR-segment changes are relative to the baseline formed by the **T-P segment.** The degree of ST elevation is typically modest (0.5 – 1m).

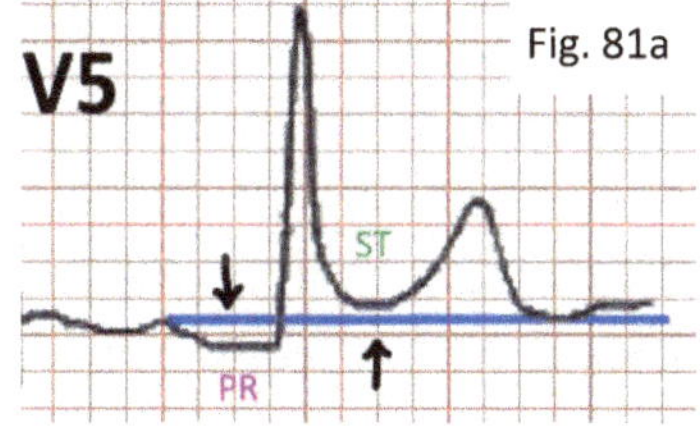

Fig. 81a

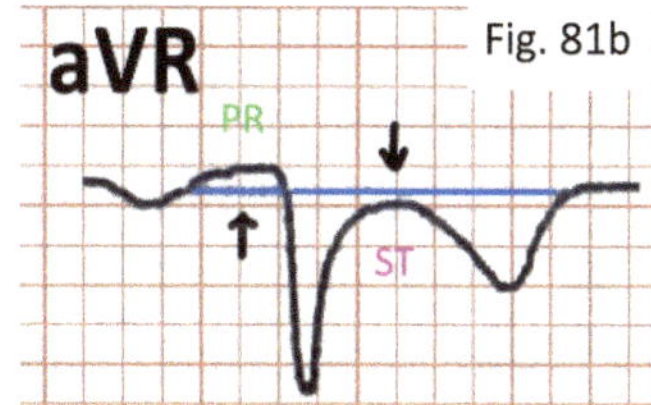

Fig. 81b

PR depression and ST elevation in V₅. Reciprocal PR elevation and ST depression in aVR

<u>Stages of Pericarditis</u>
Pericarditis is typically progress in four stages, as scribe in ECG:

Stage 1 – <u>widespread</u> STE and PR depression with reciprocal changes in aVR (occurs during the first two weeks)
Stage 2 – normalization of ST changes; generalized T wave flattening (1 to 3 weeks)
Stage 3 – flattened T waves become inverted (3 to numerous weeks)
Stage 4 – ECG returns to normal (several weeks onwards)

NB: Less than 50% of patients progress through all four classical stages and evolution of changes may not follow this typical pattern.

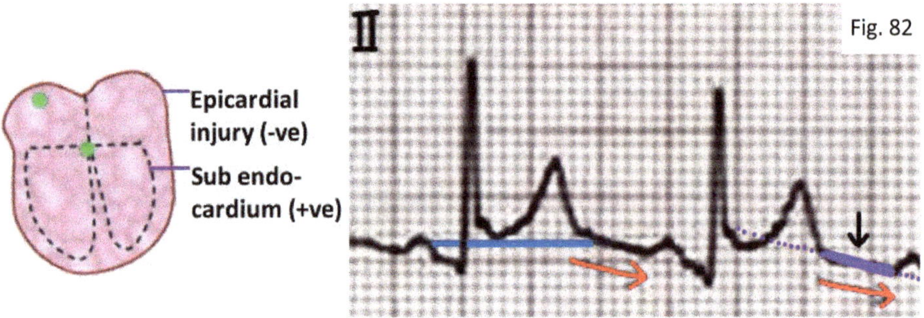

On first viewing there is obvious ST elevation and PR depression; however, lets apply the true base line which is the TP line. Applying the TP-line as base line now, there is neither PR depression nor ST elevation. The down sloping TP line is called **Spodick's** sign.

Acute Pericarditis:
- Sinus tachycardia
- Widespread concave STE and PR depression (I, II, III, aVF, V₄₋₆)
- Reciprocal ST depression and PR elevation in V1 and aVR
- **Spodick's** sign best visualized in lead II

Pericarditis vs Benign Early Repolarization

Pericarditis can be difficult to differentiate from Benign Early Repolarization (BER) as both conditions are associated with concave ST elevation. One useful trick to distinguish between these two entities is to look at the ST-segment / T wave ratio and the *"Fishhook"* pattern.

ST-segment / T wave ratio:

- The vertical height of the ST segment elevation (from the end of the PR segment to the J point) is measured and compared to the amplitude of the T wave in V_6.
- A ratio of > 0.25 suggests pericarditis
- A ratio of < 0.25 suggests BER (Benign Early Repolarization)

Fig. 83a

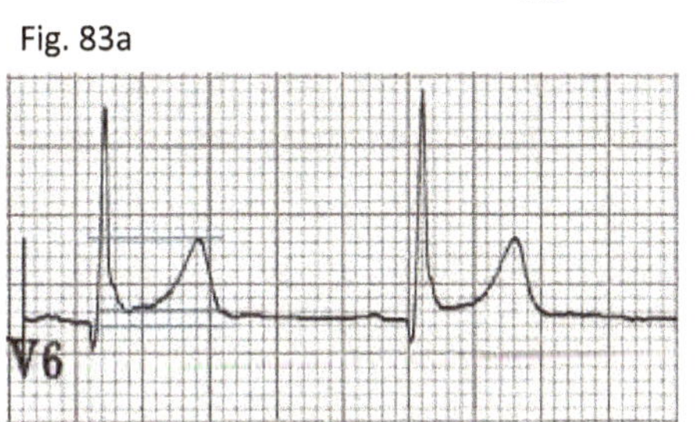

Fig. 83b

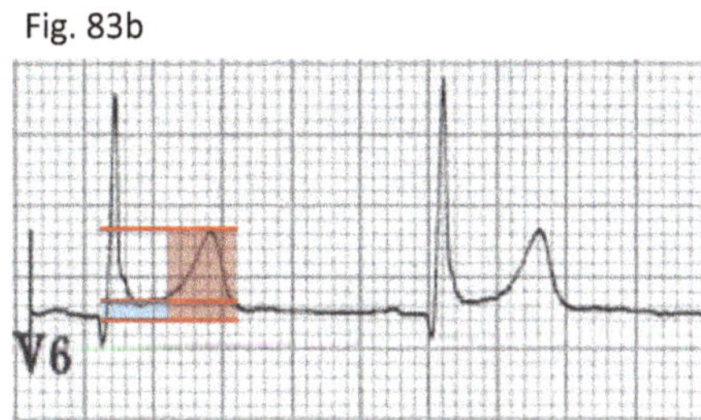

Benign Early Repolarization

- ST segment height = 1 mm
- T wave height = 6 mm
- ST / T wave ratio = 0.16
- The ST / T wave ratio < 0.25 is consistent with BER.

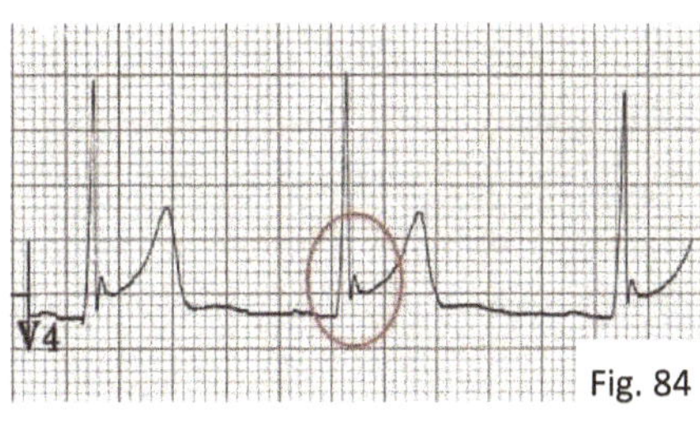

Fig. 84

Another clue that suggests BER is the presence of a notched or irregular J point: the so-called *"fishhook"* pattern. This is often best seen in lead V4.

Notched J-point elevation in V_4 with a "fishhook" morphology, characteristic of BER.

Pericarditis vs STEMI

Classic teaching of generalized concave up ST elevation and PR elevation in aVR is **not** dependable for distinguishing pericarditis from ST elevation myocardial infarction (STEMI).

- Pericarditis can cause localized ST elevation but there should be no reciprocal ST depression (except in aVR and V_1).
- STEMI, like pericarditis, can also cause concave up ST elevation.
- Only STEMI causes convex up or horizontal ST elevation.
- ST elevation greater in III than II strongly suggests a STEMI.
- PR segment depression is only reliably seen in viral pericarditis, not by other causes. It is often only an early transient phenomenon (lasting only hours). MI can also cause PR segment depression due to atrial infarction (or PR segment elevation in aVR).
- You cannot rely on history either — STEMI can also cause positional or pleuritic pain. A pericardial friction rub is also audible.

Look for features of STEMI primarily:
- Search for ST depression in leads other than aVR and V_1
- Look for ST elevation in lead III > II
- Search for horizontal or convex upward ST elevation

If the above absent, additional findings suggestive pericarditis include:

- PR depression in multiple leads. This is *suggestive* of pericarditis, however 12% of patients with STEMI have associated PR depression
- Spodick's sign

Get serial ECGs on any patient with chest pain

...things may become more obvious with time!

With a large effusion, heart may swim freely → 'electrical alternans' occur, i.e., all the axes' changes beat to beat, and ECG scribes beat to beat varying amplitudes (see wondering atrial pacemaker).

PULMONARY DISORDER

COPD:

Emphysema produces, Enhanced residual volume, over inflated lungs.

i) Dampening effect → low voltage ECG

ii) Tubular heart → right axis deviation

iii) Pulmonary hypertension → Pressure overload → RVH → RAD

COPD also led to 'Chronic cor-pulmonale' and right sided CCF → RAH → 'P pulmonale' and RVH with repolarization abnormality.

Acute Pulmonary Embolism:

If minor, have no effect in ECG, at most it may show sinus tachycardia. But if severe, distinguishable changes scribe in ECG:

i) Acute RV dilation → RVH pattern with repolarization abnormality

ii) RBBB

iii) S1Q3 pattern ('Large S' in I and deep Q in III) [cf. in Inferior MI, at least two inferior leads show 'deep Q']

iv) Various tachyarrhythmia; especially sinus tachycardia and atrial fibrillation

Athletes' heart

Athletes or commandos undergo endurance training which alters electrophysiology massively and scribe several ominous looking indications at their ECG, though very normal and benign too.

i) The commonest is resting sinus bradycardia (even < 30 bpm) due to increased vagal tone

ii) Nonspecific ST-segment elevation in precordial leads with T wave flattening and even inversion (see 'digitalis effect') V_1 to V_4

iii) Biventricular hypertrophy

iv) Arrythmia like wandering atrial pacemaker

v) 1° or Mobitz type-I (Wenckebach) AV block

vi) Notched QRS in V_1

None of these are of any concern but frequently absolute unnecessary interventions are made, just due to unfamiliarity with these facts.

SLEEP DISORDERS

Want of adequate sleep hypoxia → tiredness, sleepy during functional hours → sleep apnea and restless leg syndrome at night → transient but chronic hypoxia → eventually develop atrial and ventricular arrhythmias and heart block, prinzmetal angina, hypertension, heart failure and myocardial infarction.

ECG during sleep of the sleep apnea patient scribes, sinus bradycardia and 1° AV block.

SUDDEN CARDIAC DEATH

Commonest cause of sudden cardiac death is CAD triggering infarction and / or ominous arrhythmia.

Other causes are:

HOCM

Long QT-interval syndrome (rarely short QT syndrome)
Cardiomyopathy (arrhythmogenic right ventricular dysplasia)
WPW syndrome

Viral myocarditis

Infiltrative diseases of myocardium (amyloidosis and sarcoidosis)
Valvular heart disease
Drug abuse (cocaine, amphetamines, etc.)
Commotio cordis (sudden blow to chest → Ventricular fibrillation

Anomalous origin of coronary arteries, which during high demand entrapped between forcefully contracting myocardium → Ventricular fibrillation.

Brugada's syndrome (genetic mutation affecting voltage gated sodium channels scribe in ECG as: RBBB with ST-segment elevation in $V_1 - V_3$. This state usually triggers polymorphic ventricular tachycardia like torsade de pointes and sadly occurs in sleep. Implantable defibrillator is the only treatment of choice as beta-blocker have no effect! Being genetic, blood related family members should be screened.

Type 1

- Coved ST segment elevation >2mm in >1 of V_1-V_3 followed by a negative T wave.
- This is the only ECG abnormality that is ***potentially*** diagnostic.
- It is often referred to as **Brugada sign**.

This ECG abnormality ***must*** be associated with one of the following ***clinical criteria*** to make the diagnosis:

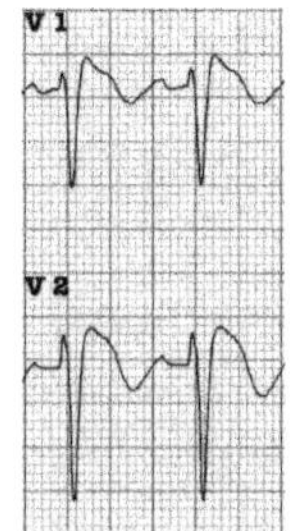

Fig. 85a

- Documented ventricular fibrillation (VF) or polymorphic ventricular tachycardia (VT)
- Family history of sudden cardiac death at <45 years old
- Coved-type ECGs in family members
- Inducibility of VT with programmed electrical stimulation
- Syncope
- Nocturnal agonal respiration

Type 2

Brugada type 2 has >2mm of saddleback shaped ST elevation.

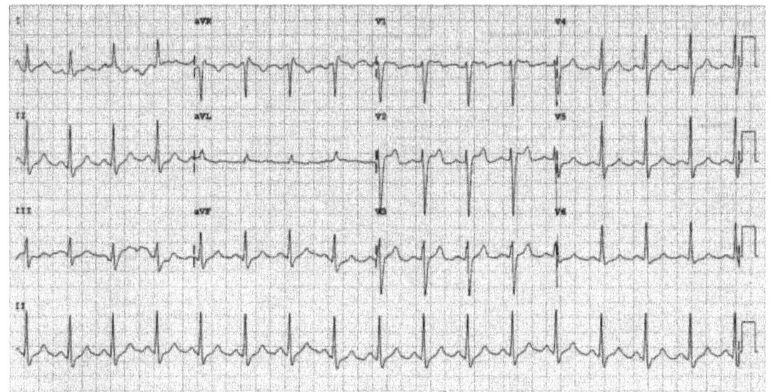

Fig. 85b

Type 3

Brugada type 3: can be the morphology of either type 1 or type 2, but with <2mm of ST segment elevation.

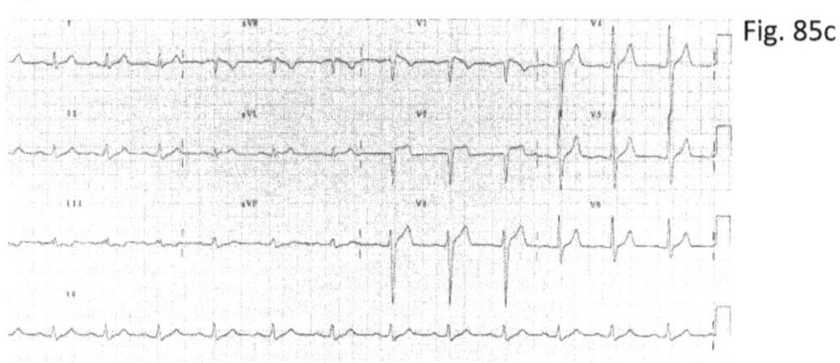

Fig. 85c

Kounis Syndrome

Acute coronary syndrome in the scenery of allergic or anaphylactic responses, generally secondary to allergic coronary vasospasm. It is also known as "allergic angina," "allergic myocardial infarction" or "coronary hypersensitivity disorder." Though the vasospastic changes seen in Kounis syndrome do not always lead to infarction. Can be induced by conditions like drugs, environmental exposures, foods, and even coronary stents; most common recognized triggers are antibiotics (28%) and insect bites (23%). It affects the cerebral and mesenteric arteries too.

Case example - (Memon et. al.):

75-year-old man with known DM-II, HTN, and hyperlipidemia presents to ER with dysuria and fever. IV Ceftriaxone was run for assumed urosepsis, which instantly developed a generalized erythematous macular rash, hypotension, and tachycardia followed by pulseless electrical activity and cardiac arrest. IV adrenaline was administered as per ALS protocol and the ECG below taken post-ROSC:

Fig. 86

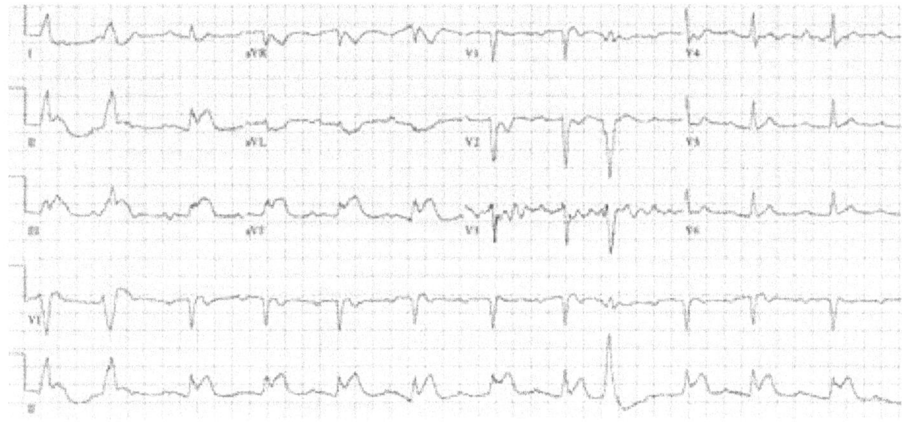

⑧ LET'S SUM UP!

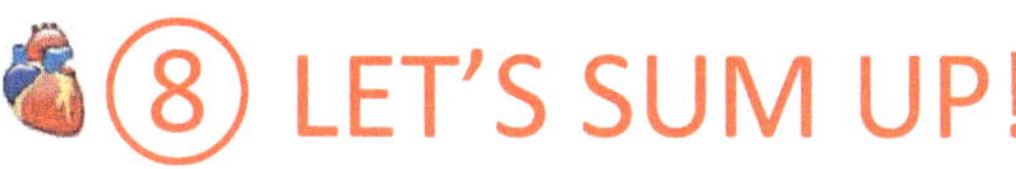

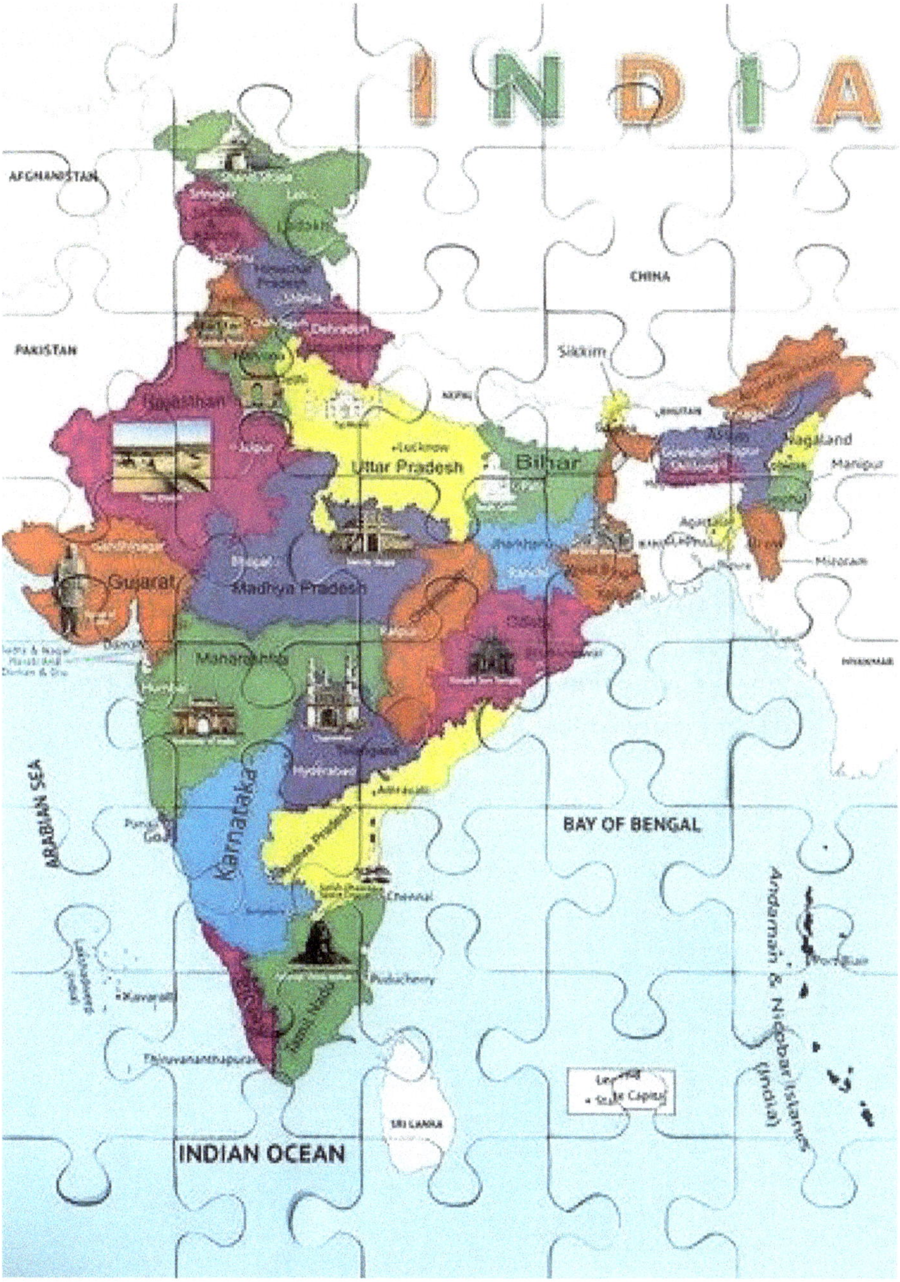
INDIA
AFGHANISTAN
PAKISTAN
CHINA
Sikkim
Dehradun
Rajasthan
Jaipur
Lucknow
Uttar Pradesh
Bihar
Assam
Nagaland
Manipur
Mizoram
Gujarat
Madhya Pradesh
MYANMAR
ARABIAN SEA
Karnataka
BAY OF BENGAL
Chennai
Puducherry
Tamil Nadu
SRI LANKA
INDIAN OCEAN
Andaman & Nicobar Islands
(India)

9 steps to REALIZE ECG

"Treat the patient – not the disease." Assess the patient clinically and make sure, the ECG is properly standardized, then follow ……

  I.   RATE: Find out heart rate
  II.   INTERVALS: Length of PR and QT intervals + width of QRS
  III. AXIS: Find all axes of P, QRS complex and T wave
  IV. RHYTHM: 4 factors to consider →
       a. P wave: morphology
       b. QRS complex: wide / narrow
       c. P wave & QRS complex: relationship
       d. Rhythm: regular / irregular
  V.   CONDUCTION BLOCKS
       a. AV block
       b. BBB and Hemiblocks
  VI. PREEXCITATION
  VII. HYPERTROPHY and DILATION
  VIII. CORONARY ARTERY DISEASE: Q waves, ST segment and T wave
  IX. OTHER CONDITIONS

I. RATE:

- Get an 'R wave' falls or almost falls at, one of the thick lines.
- Count the number of large squares (L) until the next 'R wave.'
- If the next 'R wave' does not fall at thick line, count small squares (s) to get it.
- Now, the Heart rate = $\dfrac{1500}{(L \times 5) + s}$ beat per minute (bpm).

II. INTERVALS:

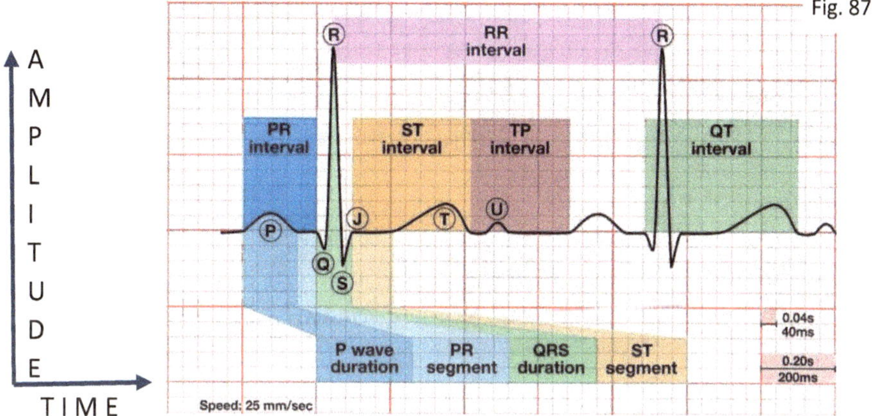

Fig. 87

III. AXIS:

	Lead I	Lead aVF
Normal	+	+
LAD*	+	-
RAD*	-	+
EAD	-	-

Note: Normal axis is -30° to +100°.

So, in case if the normal axis passing between 0° to -30° or +90° to + 100°. Then Lead aVF and Lead I will show a little bit negative.

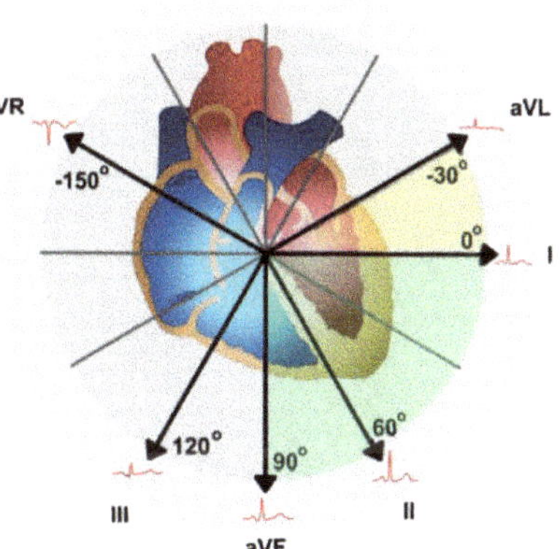

Fig. 88

IV. RHYTHM: Arrhythmia may of various origin
   1. Sinus origin
   2. Ectopic
   3. Recurrent
   4. Conduction blocks
   5. Preexcitation

Interpreting normal cardiac rhythm must be based on sign of four!

   1. Presence of normal P waves
   2. QRS-complex duration is narrow (< 0.12 seconds)
   3. Relationship between P wave & QRS (one P for every QRS)
   4. Rhythm is regular --- if any point not fulfilled, it is an arrhythmia

Rhythms of sinus origin:

1. Normal sinus rhythm

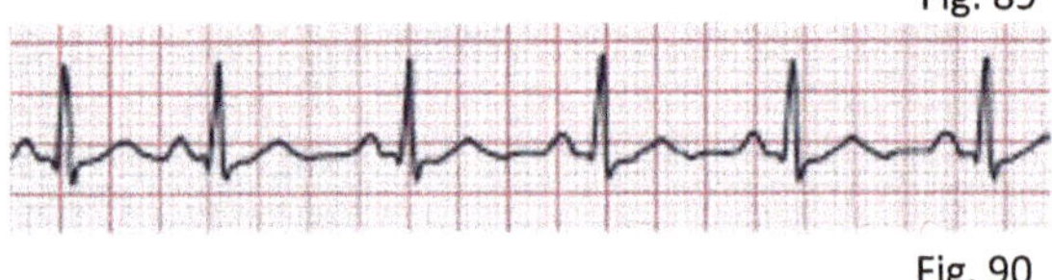

Fig. 89

2. Sinus tachycardia

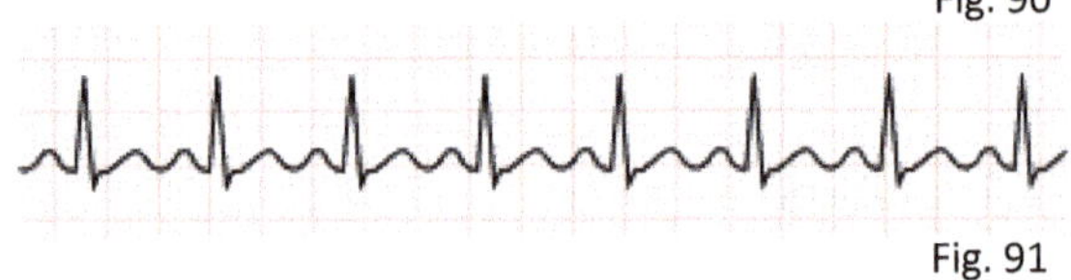

Fig. 90

3. Sinus bradycardia

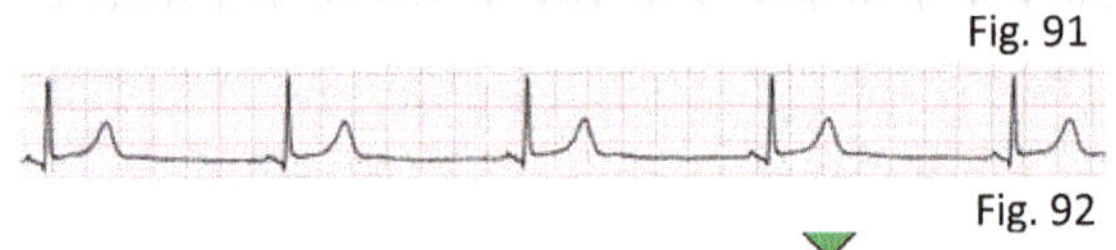

Fig. 91

4. Sinus arrest

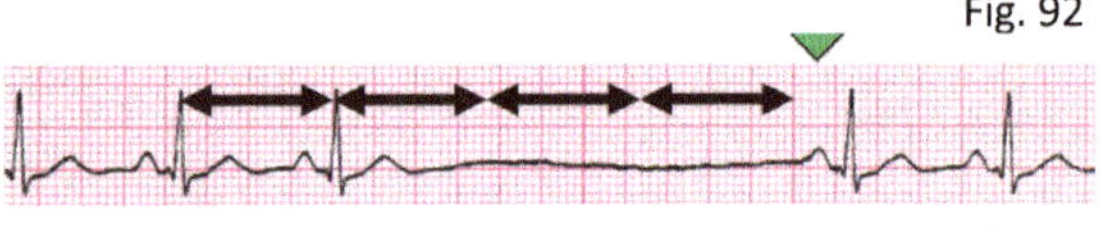

Fig. 92

5. Sinus exit block

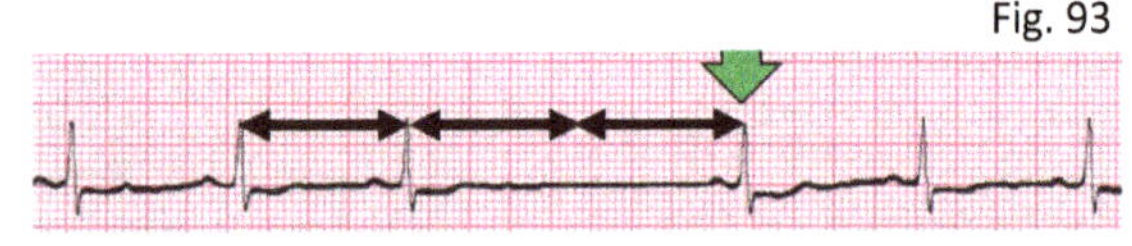

Fig. 93

6. Sinus arrest or exit block with junctional escape

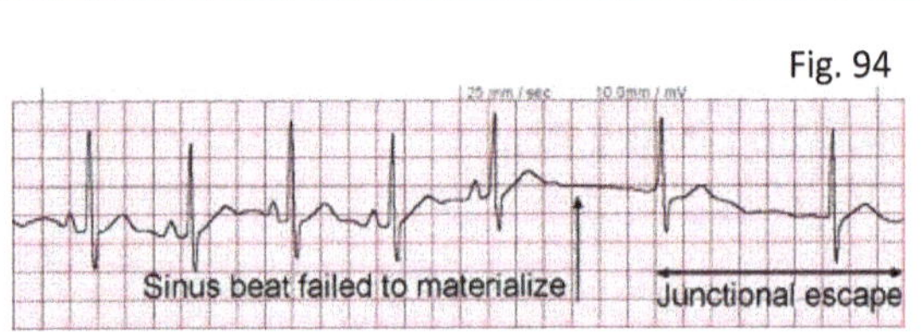

Fig. 94

Supraventricular arrhythmia:

1.	Atrial flatter	<ul><li>Regular, saw toothed</li><li>Atrial rate: 250-350</li><li>2:1, 3:1, etc. block</li><li>Ventricular rate: 1/2, 1/3, etc. of atrial rate</li><li>Carotid massage:</li><li>increases block</li></ul>
2.	Atrial fibrillation	<ul><li>Irregular, undulating baseline</li><li>Atrial rate: 350-500</li><li>Ventricular rate:</li><li>unpredictable</li></ul>
3.	Paroxysmal atrial tachycardia	<ul><li>Regular</li><li>Rate: 100-200</li><li>Characteristic automated warmup period</li><li>Carotid massage:</li><li>may slow a little</li></ul>
4.	Multifocal atrial tachycardia	<ul><li>Irregular, undulating baseline</li><li>At least 3 different P wave morphologies</li><li>Rate: Usually 100-200; if < 100 bpm – Wandering Atrial Pacemaker</li><li>Carotid massage:</li><li>no effect</li></ul>
5.	AV nodal reentrant tachycardia	<ul><li>Regular</li><li>Retrograde P (if visible)</li><li>Rate: 150-250</li><li>Carotid massage:</li><li>slows or terminates event</li></ul>
6.	AV reciprocating tachycardia	<ul><li>Regular / irregular</li><li>Rate: may very fast</li><li>QRS – may be wide / narrow</li><li>Found in WPW / LGL</li></ul>

V. CONDUCTION BLOCKS:

<u>AV Blocks:</u>

1° AV BLOCK: With every 'P' there is a 'QRS' but PR interval > 0.2 sec.

2° HEART BLOCK – MI (Mobitz type-I) :
- Every 'P' not always followed by 'QRS'.
- Progressive increase of PR interval, then a 'P' is not followed by 'QRS; then recycles.

2° HEART BLOCK – MII (Mobitz type-II) :
- Every 'P' not always followed by 'QRS'.
- PR interval stable (normal or prolonged). Some 'P' is not followed by 'QRS' as drop beat.

3° HEART BLOCK / COMPLETE : Complete dissociation between atria & ventricles. Both depolarize individually at their own rate.

<u>Bundle Branch Blocks:</u>

RBBB: 1. QRS > 0.12 seconds
2. RSR' pattern in V_1 V_2 – 'RABBIT EAR'; / tall and broad R wave
3. ST- segment depression and T wave inversion
4. Reciprocal changes in I, aVL, V_5 and V_6

LBBB: 1. QRS > 0.12 seconds
2. Broad and notched R wave + long upstroke in I, aVL, V_5 & V_6
3. Reciprocal changes in V_1 and V_2
4. LAD may be there

<u>Hemiblocks:</u>

LAHB: 1. Normal QRS duration and no ST-T changes
2. LAD (where other causes of LAD absent)

LPHB: 1. Normal QRS duration and no ST-T changes
2. RAD (where other causes of RAD absent)

<u>Bifascicular blocks</u>:

RBBB + LAHB: 1. QRS > 0.12 seconds

2. RSR' pattern in V_1 & V_2

3. LAD

RBBB + LPHB: 1. QRS > 0.12 seconds

2. RSR' pattern in V_1

3. RAD

VI. PREEXCITATION

WPW   : 1. PR interval < 0.12 seconds

2. QRS > 0.12 seconds

3. Delta wave in some leads

LGL   : 1. PR interval < 0.12 seconds

2. QRS < 0.12 seconds

3. Delta wave absent

VII. HYPERTROPHY and DILATION

Atrial Enlargement / hypertrophy:

RAE: 1. Increased amplitude of first part

2. No change in duration

3. Occasional, RAD of P wave

LAE: 1. Occasional, increased amplitude of end part

2. Increased in duration

Ventricular Hypertrophy / enlargement:

RVH: 1. RAD > + 100°

2. R:S wave amplitude in V_1 >1 and in V_6 <1

LVH: There are many criteria, the more it fulfils, more confirmatory.

1. R wave amplitude in aVL and S wave amplitude in V_3 exceeds 20 mm for women and 28 mm for men

2. R wave amplitude in V_5 / V_6 and S wave amplitude in V_1 / V_2 exceeds 35 mm

3. R wave amplitude in V_5 > 26 mm

4. R wave amplitude in V_6 > 18 mm

5. R wave amplitude in V_6 > V_5

6. R wave amplitude in I > 13 mm

7. R wave amplitude in aVF > 20 mm

8. R wave amplitude in aVL > 11 mm

9. R wave amplitude in I and S wave amplitude in III > 25 mm

♥ In all LVH, no. 1 is most accurate, and no. 2 is commonly used.

VIII.   CORONARY ARTERY DISEASE: Q waves, ST segment and T wave

MI is confirmed with history, clinical findings, cardiac markers, and sequential ECGs. In acute STEMI ECG evolves in three stages (fig. 71, 72).

Stage-I   : T wave peaking later inversion – though all T inversion is not ominous, it normally found in V_1 to V_3 in children and persist later; isolated T inversion in III also common normal finding.

Stage-II : ST-segment elevation criteria for ischemia (c.f. J-point elevation), STE must present is two closest leads.

Leads with STE	Men < 40	Men > 40	Women all ages
V_2 / V_3	> 2.5 mm	> 2 mm	> 1.5 mm
All other leads	> 1 mm	> 1 mm	> 1 mm

Stage-III : Appearance of Q waves – Ischemic Q waves never confined to single lead.

Criteria for considerable Q waves

6. Q wave > 0.04 seconds
7. Q wave depth ≥ $1/3^{rd}$ of the height of the R wave in same complex
3. Do not evaluate Q wave of aVR

Criteria for non-Q wave Infarctions

1. T wave inversion
2. ST-segment depression persist > 48 hours in proper protocol

Localizing the Infarct

<u>Anterior infarction</u>: any of the precordial leads (V_1 to V_6)

- Often caused by occlusion of the LADA
- Reciprocal changes in inferior leads
- Special T wave changes
  'De Winter' T waves – The patient with chest pain, upsloping ST depression preceding into tall symmetric T wave may be the first sign of an anterior infarction.
  Wellens' waves – Biphasic T waves in V_2 or V_3 (rarely V_4) may predict an imminent proximal LAD occlusion and an anterior infarction.

<u>Posterior infarction</u>: reciprocal changes in lead V_1 (ST-segment depression, tall R wave, which is often > the S wave in amplitude)

- Often caused by occlusion of the RCA
- Usually seen along with inferior infarctions
- ECG with posterior chest wall leads need to confirm (see fig. 76)

<u>Inferior infarction</u>: leads II, III, and aVF

- Often caused by occlusion of the RCA or its descending branch.
- Reciprocal changes in anterior and left lateral leads. T wave inversion in aVL is the commonest reciprocal change, which may appear before ST elevation and T wave inversion in inferior leads.

<u>Lateral infarction</u>: leads I, aVL, V_5 & V_6
- Often caused by occlusion of the left circumflex artery
- Reciprocal changes in inferior leads

<u>Right ventricular infarction</u>: ST elevation in V_1, often ST depression in V_2
- Virtually always along with inferior infarction. Doubt right ventricular infarction if ST elevation in III > II in amplitude
- Validate with right chest wall leads

> Note: Appearance of a new LBBB may indicate infarction.

IX. OTHER CONDITIONS

<u>Electrolyte Disturbances</u>:

Hyperkalemia: The great imitator; development of peaked T waves, PR prolongation, P wave flattening, and QRS widening. Ultimately, the QRS complexes and T waves merge to form a sine wave (a right-ward axis in the patient with wide QRS complexes suggests possible hyperkalemia as the cause); conduction blocks can develop; ultimately, asystole and ventricular fibrillation may occur.

Hypokalemia: ST depression, T wave flattening, U waves; may cause SVT and VT; if severe, QT interval prolonged.

Hypercalcemia: Shortened QT interval.

Hypocalcemia: Prolonged QT interval.

Hypomagnesemia: Prolonged QT interval.

<u>Hypothermia</u>:

Osborn waves, prolonged intervals, sinus bradycardia, slow junctional rhythm, and atrial fibrillation. Be cautious of muscle tremor artifact.

<u>Drugs</u>:

Digitalis: Therapeutic levels effect with ST-segment and T wave changes in leads with tall R waves; toxic levels effect as tachyarrhythmia and conduction blocks. PAT with block is extremely characteristic.

Drugs that can prolong QT interval: Psychotropic drugs including selective serotonin reuptake inhibitors, antifungal medications, tricyclic antidepressants, antihistamines, etc. grapefruit juice inhibits cytochrome P^{450} and results in higher drug levels and QT prolongation.

Other Cardiac Disorders:

Pericarditis – diffuse ST-segment and T wave changes; no Q waves; PR depression. A large effusion can cause low voltage, electrical alternans and wandering pacemaker.

Hypertrophic cardiomyopathy – ventricular hypertrophy, LAD, deep and narrow Q waves laterally and inferiorly.

Myocarditis – conduction blocks.

Atrial septal defect – 1° AV block, atrial tachyarrhythmia, incomplete RBBB and RAD; crochetage (small notch in R wave in limb leads), diagnosis of ASD increased to 92-100% when associated with an incomplete RBBB pattern, or when present in all three inferior leads.

Pulmonary Disorders:

Chronic obstructive pulmonary disease – Low voltage, RAD, poor R wave progression. Chronic cor-pulmonale can produce P pulmonale and RVH with repolarization abnormalities.

Acute pulmonary embolism – RVH with strain, RBBB, and S1Q3 (T3); T wave inversion in right precordial leads. Sinus tachycardia and atrial fibrillation are the most common arrhythmias.

Central Nervous System Disease:

Diffuse T wave inversion, with T waves usually wide with deep U waves.

💔 Causes of Lethal Arrhythmias and Sudden Death

Coronary artery disease, Congenital cardiac anomaly, Valvular heart disease, Trauma to the heart (commotio cordis), HOCM, Arrhythmogenic right ventricular cardiomyopathy, Viral myocarditis, Long QT syndrome, Wolff-Parkinson-White syndrome, Drug abuse (notably stimulants), Brugada syndrome, and rarely some other.

---- : : ----

Practice makes perfect. After a long time of practicing, our work will become natural, skillful, swift, and steady.

– Bruce Lee

Index not provided intentionally, to encourage go thorough again!